I0492328

Evidence Based
Therapeutic Effects of Yoga

Scientific evidence expounding the beneficial effects of yoga in over 50 medical conditions

Shashi K. Agarwal, MD

Also by the author:

- 101 Heart Healthy Lifestyles
  (co-authored with Neil K. Agarwal, MD)

- Negative Notions Positive Potions
  (co-authored with Michael E. Bowman, MSW)

- Emotional Positivity

First Edition

Disclaimer

This book is an objective review of the evidence based medical benefits of yoga. Yogic practices are only complimentary and do not replace mainstream therapeutic regimens. If you have any significant medical issues that prevents you from performing yoga or if you have discomfort doing them – please seek medical permission or advice before embarking on or continuing a self-directed yoga program. Readers should be aware that knowledge of medicine is constantly evolving. This book is not intended as a substitute for the medical advice of your physicians or other trained health care professional.

Do not disregard professional medical advice or delay seeking it because of something you have read in this book. Do not embark on any treatment change without seeking your health care provider's advice. It is a clinician's responsibility, relying on their experience and knowledge of their patients, to determine the best plan of care.

Reviewing or following information contained in this book, does not constitute a physician-patient relationship. The author and publisher accept no liability for any injury arising out of the use of material contained herein, and make no warranty, express or implied, with respect to the contents of this publication.

Printed in the USA

ISBN -13: 978-1983936364

ISBN-10: 1983936367

Copyright © 2018 Shashi K. Agarwal, MD

All rights reserved, including the right of reproduction in whole or in part in any form.

Dedicated to
The worldwide yoga community

CONTENTS

CONTENTS

Introduction: Yoga and Health

"Yoga teaches us to cure what need not be endured

and endure what cannot be cured."

B.K.S Iyengar

Yoga has become extremely popular in the United States. According to the National Center for Complimentary and Integrative Health[1], 9.5% of U.S. adults (21 million) practiced yoga and 3.1% of U.S. children (1.7 million) practiced yoga in 2016. This is a significant increase from 5.1% adults using it in 2002 and 6.1% adults using it in 2007. The number of clubs offering yoga has also been growing. In 1997, only 400,000 health clubs offered yoga classes, but in 2002, over 1.2 million health clubs offered yoga classes[2].

Yoga is extremely old – it has probably been around for 5000 years. About 1700 years ago, Pantanjali, described eight limbs of yoga, in 'Yoga sūtras', a text on Yoga theory and practice[3]. These are:

- **Yama** – Morality. Yamas are further classified into five limbs:

    - *Ahimsa*: nonviolence toward all living things. Kindness and compassion to all.
    - *Satya*: being truthful – being always transparent.
    - *Asteya*: non-stealing. You do not mentally or physically take something that is not yours.
    - *Brahmacharya*: celibacy – or proper use of energy
    - *Aparigraha*: the virtue of non-possessiveness, non-grasping or non-greediness. It also encompasses non-attachment.

- **Niyama** – Personal observances – these are also five in number:

- o *Sauca*: outer and inner cleanliness. This includes physical as well as mental cleanliness.
- o *Santosa*: contentment – finding happiness in whatever we have. Not longing for what we do not have.
- o *Tapas*: discipline – in life and especially during yoga.
- o *Svadhyaya*: self-inquiry, self-realization. Becoming aware of one's limitations.
- o *Isvarapranidhana*: establishing spirituality – a connection with a higher power.

- **Asana** – Body movement, physical postures
- **Pranayama** – Control of 'prana' (prana = cosmic energy) through controlled breathing
- **Pratyahara** – Sense control through sensory withdrawal
- **Dharana** – Concentration of the mind
- **Dhyana** – Meditation
- **Samadhi** – Union with the divine

Different 'types' of yoga, breathing exercises and meditations are all based and derived from the Pantanjali's eight limbs of yoga. In the West, the practice of yoga usually involves asanas (postures). Pranayama (breathing exercises) and Dhyana (meditation). Progressive relaxation and lectures on yoga philosophy are sometimes incorporated.

More than two-thirds of yoga practitioners reported that yoga improved their overall health. Nearly, two-thirds reported that because of practicing yoga they were motivated to exercise more regularly, and 4 in 10 reported they were motivated to eat healthier. More than 80 percent of yoga users reported reduced stress with yoga[2]. Most felt better – they reported a greater sense of relaxation, improved body-image and self-confidence, increased attentiveness, enhanced efficiency, lower irritability, improved interpersonal relationships, and a more positive and optimistic outlook on life.

Yoga has also garnered intense scientific scrutiny. Research studies on yoga and medical conditions published in 2013 were three times as high as in 2010[5]. Research continues to proliferate[6]. The most common research publications on yoga and medical conditions were related to breast cancer, depression, asthma, and type 2 diabetes mellitus[7]. There were also significant number of studies on low back pain and hypertension.

Yoga is a multimodal practice[8] and all clinical studies have used different yoga styles, yoga postures and breathing techniques in their intervention groups. Some included yoga meditation, relaxation and lectures on yogic philosophy. Besides the therapeutic benefits noted in specific conditions, yoga has also demonstrated a major benefit on improving the quality of life of patients[9]. Most of the emerging data is painting a favorable picture of yoga as a feasible adjunct therapeutic modality in several common diseases.

A growing body of research evidence supports the belief that the multimodal yoga techniques, usually done together, improve physical and mental health parameters, through complicated anatomic-physiological mechanisms. The different components of yoga – asanas, pranayama, meditation and relaxation all appear to contribute to the overall positive effects, in most cases. Some of the benefits and involved biological mechanisms include:

- There is an improvement in the strength (especially of the core muscles) and flexibility[10]. Endurance is enhanced[11]. Balance[12] and co-ordination is improved[13].
- Respiratory parameters, such as forced vital capacity (FVC), forced expiratory volume during the first second (FEV1), FEV1/FVC ratio, forced expiratory volume during the middle one half of the FVC (FEV 25-75%), peak expiratory flow rate, maximum voluntary ventilation and slow vital capacity, improve[14-17]. The muscles of respiration are strengthened[18].
- There is an improvement in cardiovascular parameters. There is a decrease in blood pressure[19]. and peripheral arterial resistance[20]. Lipid profile is improved[21]. There is an increase in ejection fraction[22], cardiac output [23] and heart rate variability[24]. There is a decrease in coronary atherosclerosis[25].

- There is a down-regulation of the hypothalamo pituitary adrenal (HPA) axis with decreased cortisol levels,[26,27] and increased neurotransmitter gamma-aminobutyric acid (GABA) levels[28]. Increased GABA levels help improve the mood [29,30].
- Serotonin levels are increased. (serotonin positively affects the mood)[31]. Yoga may also increase endogenous dopamine release in the ventral striatum, a major area of the brain's reward system, explaining the 'feel good' reward with yoga[32]. Oxytocin levels improve, especially in schizophrenics – oxytocin improves social cognition abilities[33].
- There is an increase in the grey matter in the prefrontal cortex (executive center)[34,35], and hippocampus (with a decrease in neuro-senescence)[36] and a decrease in the amygdala (resulting in a decrease in anxiety and fear)[37]. Executive function, including cognition is improved[38,39]. There is more self-awareness and self-regulation. Neuroplasticity within the brain, especially between the basal ganglia, thalamus and cortex occurs, allowing for a better top-down control.
- Meditation helps reduce mind wandering and negative rumination. There is an increased self-compassion and self-transcendence. Meditation practices have also been shown to increase melatonin levels[40] and improve cognitive processes[41].
- Sympathetic activity is decreased. Levels of plasma epinephrine and norepinephrine (catecholamines secreted from adrenal medulla) are decreased following yogic practice[42].
- Parasympathetic activity is increased[43-46]. This increase in parasympathetic activity, primarily with vagus stimulation, improves the bottom-up control.
- Biomarkers of inflammation are reduced[47-49]. Inflammation is a critical factor behind the development and progression of atherosclerosis[50] and possibly cancer[51].
- There is an increase in the left insular grey and white matter, with yoga practice. This correlates with increased pain tolerance[52]. Immune function is also improved[53].

- Overall quality of life is improved[54].

The common drawback in most studies is the small number of participants, the short duration of the study and often the lack of proper design. However, encouraged by the positive results of these studies, more robust trials are being implemented. In the coming years, the therapeutic role of yoga in many conditions will become clearer and more objectively supported by clinical evidence, allowing yoga to be included in several guidelines aimed at disease management.

Yoga is simple and easy to do. It can be practiced in a non-secular way[55]. It can be done by all communities, irrespective of the race or income[56,57]. It is non-pharmacological and non-surgical. It can be individually tailored. It is cheap (compared to pharmaceutical/surgical interventions and when done at home). Serious side effects are rare[58]. It can be done almost anywhere and at any time. Its practice is possible in all age groups[59,60]. Adherence is good and attrition rate is low[61]

Increasing scientific evidence, as detailed in this book, also confirms its feasibility in most medical conditions.

References

1. nccih.nih.gov/research/statistics/NHIS/2012/mind-body/yoga – accessed 1/20/18.
2. Barnes P, Bloom B, Nahin R. Complementary and alternative medicine use among adults and children: United States, 2007. Natl Health Stat Report. 2008. December 10;(12):1–23.
3. Woods, James Haughton (1914). the Yoga-system of Patañjali: or, the ancient Hindu doctrine of Concentration of Mind Embracing the Mnemonic Rules, called Yoga-sūtras, of Patañjali and the Comment, called Yoga-bhāshya, attributed to Veda-Vyāsa and the Explanation, called Tattvaiçāradī, of Vāchaspati-miçra. Cambridge, MA: Harvard University Press.
4. Stussman BJ, Black LI, Barnes PM, Clarke TC, Nahin RL. Wellness-related use of common complementary health approaches among adults: United States, 2012. National health statistics reports; no 85. Hyattsville, MD: National Center for Health Statistics. 2015.
5. Cramer H, Lauche R, Dobos G. Characteristics of randomized controlled trials of yoga: a bibliometric analysis. BMC Complementary and Alternative Medicine. 2014;14:328. doi:10.1186/1472-6882-14-328.

6. Sherman KJ. Guidelines for developing yoga interventions for randomized trials. Evid Based Comp Alt Med. 2012:1–15.
7. Cramer H, Lauche R, Dobos G. Characteristics of randomized controlled trials of yoga: a bibliometric analysis. BMC Complementary and Alternative Medicine. 2014;14:328. doi:10.1186/1472-6882-14-328.
8. Feuerstein G. The Yoga Tradition. Prescott: Hohm Press; 1998.; De Michaelis E. A History of Modern Yoga: Patanjali and Western Esotericism. London, UK: Continuum International Publishing Group; 2005.
9. Woodyard C. Exploring the therapeutic effects of yoga and its ability to increase quality of life. Intern J Yoga 2011;4:49–54.
10. Halder K, Chatterjee A, Pal R, Tomer OS, Saha M. Age related differences of selected Hatha yoga practices on anthropometric characteristics, muscular strength and flexibility of healthy individuals. International Journal of Yoga. 2015;8(1):37-46. doi:10.4103/0973-6131.146057.
11. Lau C, Yu R, Woo J. Effects of a 12-Week Hatha Yoga Intervention on Cardiorespiratory Endurance, Muscular Strength and Endurance, and Flexibility in Hong Kong Chinese Adults: A Controlled Clinical Trial. Evidence-based Complementary and Alternative Medicine : eCAM. 2015;2015:958727. doi:10.1155/2015/958727.
12. Ulger O, Yagli NV. Effects of yoga on balance and gait properties in women with musculoskeletal problems: a pilot study. Complement Ther Clin Pract. 2011;17(1):13–15. doi: 10.1016/j.ctcp.2010.06.006.
13. B. Donahoe-Fillmore, M. Holdash, C. Moore, J. Robertson. The effect of yoga postures on balance, coordination and flexibility in typically developing children. Pediatric Physical Therapy: April 2004 - Volume 16 - Issue 1 - p 51. doi: 10.1097/01.PEP.0000115221.39160.D5.
14. Abel AN, Lloyd LK, Williams JS. The effects of regular yoga practice on pulmonary function in healthy individuals: A literature review. J Altern Complement Med. 2013;19:185–90.
15. Maheshkumar Kuppusamy, K Dilara, P Ravishankar, and A Julius. Effect of Bhrāmarī Prāṇāyāma Practice on Pulmonary Function in Healthy Adolescents: A Randomized Control Study. Anc Sci Life. 2017 Apr-Jun; 36(4): 196–199.
16. Yadav RK, Das S. Effect of yogic practice on pulmonary functions in young females. I ndian J Physiol Pharmacol. 2001 Oct;45(4):493-6.
17. Telles S, Singh N, Balkrishna A. Metabolic and Ventilatory Changes During and After High-Frequency Yoga Breathing. Medical Science Monitor Basic Research. 2015;21:161-171. doi:10.12659/MSMBR.894945.
18. Mandanmohan, Jatiya L, Udupa K, Bhavanani AB. Effect of yoga training on handgrip, respiratory pressures and pulmonary function. Indian J Physiol Pharmacol. 2003 Oct;47(4):387-92.
19. Brook R.D., Appel L.J., Rubenfire M. Beyond medications and diet. Alternative approaches to lowering blood pressure. A Scientific

Statement from American Heart Association. Hypertension.
2013;61:1360–1363.

20. Sivasankaran S, Pollard-Quintner S, Sachdeva R, Pugeda J, Hoq SM, Zarich SW. The effect of a six-week program of yoga and meditation on brachial artery reactivity: do psychosocial interventions affect vascular tone? Clin Cardiol. 2006 Sep;29(9):393-8.

21. Pal A, Srivastava N, Tiwari S, Verma NS, Narain VS, Agrawal GG, Natu SM, Kumar K. Effect of yogic practices on lipid profile and body fat composition in patients of coronary artery disease. Complement Ther Med. 2011;19:122–127.

22. Raghuram N, Parachuri VR, Swarnagowri MV, et al. Yoga based cardiac rehabilitation after coronary artery bypass surgery: One-year results on LVEF, lipid profile and psychological states – A randomized controlled study. Indian Heart Journal. 2014;66(5):490-502. doi:10.1016/j.ihj.2014.08.007.

23. Miles SC, Chun-Chung C, Hsin-Fu L, Hunter SD, Dhindsa M, Nualnim N, Tanaka H. Arterial blood pressure and cardiovascular responses to yoga practice. Altern Ther Health Med. 2013 Jan-Feb;19(1):38-45.

24. Tyagi A, Cohen M. Yoga and heart rate variability: A comprehensive review of the literature. International Journal of Yoga. 2016;9(2):97-113. doi:10.4103/0973-6131.183712.

25. Manchanda S.C., Narang R., Reddy K.S. Retardation of coronary atherosclerosis with yoga lifestyle intervention. J Assoc Physicians India. 2000;48:687–694.

26. Kamei T, Toriumi Y, Kimura H, Ohno S, Kumano H, Kimura K. Decrease in serum cortisol during yoga exercise is correlated with alpha wave activation. Percept Mot Skills. 2000;90(3 Pt 1):1027–1032.

27. Ross A, Thomas S. The health benefits of yoga and exercise: a review of comparison studies. J Altern Complement Med. 2010;16(1):3–12.

28. Streeter CC, Jensen JE, Perlmutter RM, Cabral HJ, Tian H, Terhune DB, Ciraulo DA, Renshaw PF. Yoga asana sessions increase brain GABA levels: a pilot study. J Altern Complement Med. 2007;13(4):419–426. doi: 10.1089/acm.2007.6338.

29. Streeter CC, Whitfield TH, Owen L, et al. Effects of yoga versus walking on mood, anxiety, and brain GABA levels: a randomized controlled MRS study. J Altern Complement Med. 2010;16(11):1145–1152.

30. Streeter CC, Gerbarg PL, Saper RB, et al. Effects of yoga on the autonomic nervous system, gamma-aminobutyric-acid, and allostasis in epilepsy, depression, and post-traumatic stress disorder. Med Hypotheses. 2012;78(5):571–579.

31. Pal R, Singh SN, Chatterjee A, Saha M. Age-related changes in cardiovascular system, autonomic functions, and levels of BDNF of healthy active males: role of yogic practice. Age. 2014;36(4):9683. doi:10.1007/s11357-014-9683-7.

32. Schultz W. Getting formal with dopamine and reward. Neuron. 2002;36(2):241–263.

33. Jayaram N, Varambally S, Behere RV, et al. Effect of yoga therapy on plasma oxytocin and facial emotion recognition deficits in patients of

schizophrenia. Indian Journal of Psychiatry. 2013;55(Suppl 3): S409-S413. doi:10.4103/0019-5545.116318.

34. Froeliger B, Garland EL, McClernon FJ. Yoga Meditation Practitioners Exhibit Greater Gray Matter Volume and Fewer Reported Cognitive Failures: Results of a Preliminary Voxel-Based Morphometric Analysis. Evidence-based Complementary and Alternative Medicine: eCAM. 2012;2012:821307. doi:10.1155/2012/821307.

35. Afonso RF, Balardin JB, Lazar S, et al. Greater Cortical Thickness in Elderly Female Yoga Practitioners—A Cross-Sectional Study. Frontiers in Aging Neuroscience. 2017;9:201. doi:10.3389/fnagi.2017.00201.

36. Hariprasad VR, Varambally S, Shivakumar V, Kalmady SV, Venkatasubramanian G, Gangadhar BN. Yoga increases the volume of the hippocampus in elderly subjects. Indian Journal of Psychiatry. 2013;55(Suppl 3): S394-S396. doi:10.4103/0019-5545.116309.

37. Hölzel BK, Carmody J, Evans KC, et al. Stress reduction correlates with structural changes in the amygdala. Social Cognitive and Affective Neuroscience. 2010;5(1):11-17. doi:10.1093/scan/nsp034.

38. Gard T, Hölzel BK, Lazar SW. The potential effects of meditation on age-related cognitive decline: a systematic review. Annals of the New York Academy of Sciences. 2014;1307:89-103. doi:10.1111/nyas.12348.

39. Cahn BR, Goodman MS, Peterson CT, Maturi R, Mills PJ. Yoga, Meditation and Mind-Body Health: Increased BDNF, Cortisol Awakening Response, and Altered Inflammatory Marker Expression after a 3-Month Yoga and Meditation Retreat. Frontiers in Human Neuroscience. 2017;11:315. doi:10.3389/fnhum.2017.00315.

40. Tooley GA, Armstrong SM, Norman TR, Sali A. Acute increases in Night-time plasma melatonin levels following a period of mediatation. Biol Psychol. 2000;53:69–78.

41. Zeidan F, Martucci KT, Kraft RA, McHaffie JG, Coghill RC. Neural correlates of mindfulness meditation-related anxiety relief. Social Cognitive and Affective Neuroscience. 2014;9(6):751-759. doi:10.1093/scan/nst041.

42. Pal R, Singh SN, Chatterjee A, Saha M. Age-related changes in cardiovascular system, autonomic functions, and levels of BDNF of healthy active males: role of yogic practice. Age. 2014;36(4):9683. doi:10.1007/s11357-014-9683-7.

43. Khattab K, Khattab AA, Ortak J, Richardt G, Bonnemeier H. Iyengar yoga increases cardiac parasympathetic nervous modulation among healthy yoga practitioners. Evid Based Complement Alternat Med. 2007;4:511–7.

44. Vinay A, Venkatesh D, Ambarish V. Impact of short-term practice of yoga on heart rate variability. International Journal of Yoga. 2016;9(1):62-66. doi:10.4103/0973-6131.171714.

45. Bharshankar JR, Mandape AD, Phatak MS, Bharshankar RN. Autonomic Functions in Raja-yoga Meditators. Indian J Physiol Pharmacol. 2015 Oct-Dec;59(4):396-401.

46. Bhaskar L, Kharya C, Deepak KK, Kochupillai V. Assessment of Cardiac Autonomic Tone Following Long Sudarshan Kriya Yoga in Art of Living Practitioners. J Altern Complement Med. 2017 Sep;23(9):705-712. doi: 10.1089/acm.2016.0391. Epub 2017 Jul 10.

47. Pullen PR, Nagamia SH, Mehta PK, Thompson WR, Benardot D, Hammoud R, et al. Effects of yoga on inflammation and exercise capacity in patients with chronic heart failure. J Card Fail. 2008;14(5):407–13.

48. Bower JE, Irwin MR. Mind-body therapies and control of inflammatory biology: A descriptive review. Brain, behavior, and immunity. 2016;51:1-11. doi:10.1016/j.bbi.2015.06.012.

49. Cahn BR, Goodman MS, Peterson CT, Maturi R, Mills PJ. Yoga, Meditation and Mind-Body Health: Increased BDNF, Cortisol Awakening Response, and Altered Inflammatory Marker Expression after a 3-Month Yoga and Meditation Retreat. Frontiers in Human Neuroscience. 2017;11:315. doi:10.3389/fnhum.2017.00315.

50. Rodolfo Paoletti, Antonio M. Gotto, David P. Hajjar. Inflammation in Atherosclerosis and Implications for Therapy. Circulation. 2004;109:III-20-III-26.

51. Coussens LM, Werb Z. Inflammation and cancer. Nature. 2002;420(6917):860-867. doi:10.1038/nature01322.

52. Villemure C, Čeko M, Cotton VA, Bushnell MC. Insular Cortex Mediates Increased Pain Tolerance in Yoga Practitioners. Cerebral Cortex (New York, NY). 2014;24(10):2732-2740. doi:10.1093/cercor/bht124.

53. Gopal A, Mondal S, Gandhi A, Arora S, Bhattacharjee J. Effect of integrated yoga practices on immune responses in examination stress - A preliminary study. Int J Yoga. 2011;4:26–32.

54. Woodyard C. Exploring the therapeutic effects of yoga and its ability to increase quality of life. International Journal of Yoga. 2011;4(2):49-54. doi:10.4103/0973-6131.85485.

55. https: //www.usatoday.com/story/opinion/2013/05/18/yoga-religion-column/2158377/ (accessed 1/2/18)

56. Keosaian JE, Lemaster CM, Dresner D, et al. "We're All in This Together": A Qualitative Study of Predominantly Low Income Minority Participants in a Yoga Trial for Chronic Low Back Pain. Complementary therapies in medicine. 2016;24:34-39. doi:10.1016/j.ctim.2015.11.007.

57. Firestone KA, Carson JW, Mist SD, Carson KM, Jones KD. Interest In Yoga Among Fibromyalgia Patients: An International Internet Survey. International journal of yoga therapy. 2014;24:117-124.

58. Cramer H, Krucoff C, Dobos G. Adverse events associated with yoga: a systematic review of published case reports and case series. PLoS One. 2013;8(10):e75515. doi: 10.1371/journal.pone.0075515.

59. Berger DL, Silver EJ, Stein RE. Effects of yoga on inner-city children's well-being: a pilot study. Altern Ther Health Med. 2009 Sep-Oct;15(5):36-42.

60. Chen KM, Fan JT, Wang HH, Wu SJ, Li CH, Lin HS. Silver yoga exercises improved physical fitness of transitional frail elders. Nurs Res. 2010 Sep-Oct;59(5):364-70. doi: 10.1097/NNR.0b013e3181ef37d5.

61. Flegal KE, Kishiyama S, Zajdel D, Haas M, Oken BS. Adherence to yoga and exercise interventions in a 6-month clinical trial. BMC Complement Altern Med. 2007;7:37.

Alcohol Use Disorder*

Alcohol intake is common in the American population. The 2015 National Survey on Drug Use and Health reported that amongst people ages 18 and older, 86.4 percent reported that they had imbibed alcohol at some point in their lifetime: 70.1 percent drank in the past year, and 56.0 percent had consumed it in the past month[1]. Moderate drinking - up to 1 drink per day for women and up to 2 drinks per day for men, has been found to be beneficial for health – decreased risk of heart disease, stroke and diabetes mellitus – and death[2,3]. In the United States, a standard drink contains 0.6 ounces (14.0 grams or 1.2 tablespoons) of pure alcohol. Generally, this amount of pure alcohol is also present in 12-ounces of beer (5% alcohol content), 8-ounces of malt liquor (7% alcohol content), 5-ounces of wine (12% alcohol content), or 1.5-ounces of 80-proof (40% alcohol content) distilled spirits or liquor (e.g., gin, rum, vodka, whiskey)[3].

Excessive alcohol intake includes binge drinking and heavy alcohol consumption – but may not necessarily be classified as an alcohol use disorder. Binge drinking, is defined as consuming 4 or more drinks for women and 5 or more drinks for men, during a single occasion. It is the most common form of excessive alcohol drinking[4]. Data indicates that in 2015, binge drinking was reported by 26.9 percent of people ages 18 or older in the previous month. Heavy drinking is defined as consuming 8 or more drinks for women and 15 or more drinks for men, per week[5]. Data on heavy alcohol use reveals that it is present in 7.0 percent of people aged 18 or older[6]. It is estimated that almost 16 million people (9.8 million men and 5.3 million women), ages 18 and older, suffer from alcohol use disorder (AUD) in the US[7]. Unfortunately, adolescents also have this disorder – in 2015, it affected almost 623,000 adolescents[8].

Alcohol use disorder is an inability to stop or control alcohol use despite negative consequences. According to the Diagnostics and Statistical Manual of Mental Disorders, Fifth Edition (DSM-5), published by the American Psychiatry Association, alcohol abuse and alcohol dependence. Alcohol use disorder is recognized as an alcohol related impairment with an inability to stop or control its consumption, despite adverse social, occupational or health consequences[9].

Excessive alcohol intake is harmful. It is responsible for an increased incidence of unintentional injuries such as falls, burns, drownings and car crashes, sexual and other assaults and poor academic performance[10-12]. Suicides are also common in this population[13]. Heavy alcohol intake also leads to the development of many diseases. These include high blood pressure, heart disease and stroke[14]. It can also lead to depression and anxiety[15] and social and family problems[16-17]. Alcohol is neuro-toxic and chronic alcoholism damages the brain18. Alcohol can cause several digestive problems, including diseases of the liver. Liver diseases such as cirrhosis of the liver and liver transplants are common in people with alcohol abuse[19,20]. Alcohol intake also places the individual at an increased risk of several cancers – those affecting the mouth, esophagus, pharynx, larynx, liver, colon and breast21. According to the World Health Organization, 2.5 million lives are lost worldwide every year from the harmful effects of alcohol[22].

AUD is difficult to treat[23]. Drugs recommended include naltrexone and acamprosate as first line for patients with moderate to severe AUD. Drugs suggested as a second line include topiramate and gabapentin[24]. Relapses, unfortunately, are common. It is estimated that a relapse is noted in almost 50% of treated alcohol-dependent individuals by the end of the first year[25]. Exercise[26] and meditation[27] have shown benefit in these patients – and yoga includes both modalities.

Yoga and Alcohol Use Disorder

Yoga has been considered as a complementary treatment for alcoholics, with encouraging results[28-29].

In a 90-day residential group pilot treatment program for substance abuse, 8 men who had recently undergone alcohol detoxification, symptom management and quality of recovery improved with yoga therapy[30].

In a randomized controlled trial of 60 male inpatients with alcohol dependence, patients who were randomly given Sudarshana Kriya yoga for two weeks had greater reduction of cortisol, adrenocorticotropic hormone, and biological hormones associated with stress as compared to the usual care controls[31]. Cortisol levels increase in patients with alcohol abuse – due to the activation of the hypothalamic-pituitary-adrenal axis[32]. Cortisol levels remain high after alcohol intake is stopped and during withdrawal – and may contribute to the frequent relapses[33].

In women, aged 18 to 65 years, suffering from PTSD, yoga intervention consisting of 12 Kripalu-based Hatha yoga sessions of 75 minutes each, resulted in a trend toward decreased alcohol use, when compared to the control group[34].

Meditation has also shown benefit in patients with alcohol addiction[35]. Khanna and group in a narrative report suggest that smoking dependence may be broken by generating a sense of self-awareness, self-control, and self-realization – by using a 'whole system' approach – pranayama, asana, dharana, pratyahara and dhyana. A similar approach may help break the cycle of alcohol addiction[35].

In a study involving 126 individuals who practiced transcendental meditation and 90 individuals in a matched control group, the continued use of alcohol was examined. There was no discontinuation reported in the control group, for beer or wine consumption, while the meditation group reported a 40% discontinuation within the first 6 months. After 25-39 months of meditation, 54% of the meditators reported discontinuation of hard liquor consumption, compared to only 1% in the control group[36]. Abstinence of alcohol use was also noted in another study using transcendental meditation[37].

In another study of 53 alcohol-dependent adults, mindfulness therapy significantly improved alcohol addiction automaticity and decreased stress reactivity – resulting in better awareness of the craving and increased ability to avoid alcohol in stressful situations[38].

Stress not only contributes to alcoholism[39] but also plays a role in relapse[40]. Yoga[41] and meditation[42] are good stress relieving interventions.

Conclusion

Alcohol is often abused, and many people develop dependence. Alcohol use disorder is dangerous to the health. It is difficult to prevent or cure. It is also associated with frequent relapses. Evidence based data suggests that yoga practices may help reduce heavy alcohol use and help diminish the frequent relapses.

* Adapted from: Neil K Agarwal and Shashi K Agarwal. The Role of Yoga in the Complementary Treatment of Cancer. MOJ Yoga & Physical Therapy – 2017. (printed with permission)

References

1. Substance Abuse and Mental Health Services Administration (SAMHSA). 2015 National Survey on Drug Use and Health (NSDUH). Table 2.41B—Alcohol Use in Lifetime, Past Year, and Past Month among Persons Aged 12 or Older, by Demographic Characteristics: Percentages, 2014 and 2015. Available at: https://www.samhsa.gov/data/sites/default/files/NSDUH-DetTabs-2015/NSDUH-DetTabs-2015/NSDUH-DetTabs-2015.htm#tab2-41b. Accessed 12/18/17.
2. U.S. Department of Agriculture. Scientific Report of the 2015 Dietary Guidelines Advisory Committee, Part D. Chapter 2, Table D2.3, p. 43. Available at: health.gov/dietaryguidelines/2015-scientific-report/pdfs/scientific-report-of-the-2015-dietary-guidelines-advisory-committee.pdf. Accessed 1/18/17.
3. U.S. Department of Health and Human Services and U.S. Department of Agriculture. 2015-2020 Dietary Guidelines for Americans. 8th Edition, Washington, DC; 2015.
4. cdc.gov/alcohol/fact-sheets/alcohol-use.htm - accessed 1/15/18.
5. cdc.gov/alcohol/fact-sheets/alcohol-use.htm - accessed 1/15/18.
6. Substance Abuse and Mental Health Services Administration (SAMHSA). 2015 National Survey on Drug Use and Health (NSDUH). Table 2.46B—Alcohol Use, Binge Alcohol Use, and Heavy Alcohol Use in Past Month among Persons Aged 12 or Older, by Demographic Characteristics: Percentages, 2014 and 2015.
7. (SAMHSA). 2015 National Survey on Drug Use and Health (NSDUH). Table 5.6A—Substance Use Disorder in Past Year among Persons Aged 18 or Older, by Demographic Characteristics: Numbers in Thousands, 2014 and 2015.
8. Substance Abuse and Mental Health Services Administration (SAMHSA). 2015 National Survey on Drug Use and Health (NSDUH).

Table 5.5A—Substance Use Disorder in Past Year among Persons Aged 12 to 17, by Demographic Characteristics: Numbers in Thousands, 2014 and 2015.

9. American Psychiatric Association issued the 5th edition of the Diagnostic and Statistical Manual of Mental Disorders (DSM–5).

10. Substance Abuse and Mental Health Services Administration

11. Hingson, R.W.; Zha, W.; and Weitzman, E.R. Magnitude of and trends in alcohol-related mortality and morbidity among U.S. college students ages 18–24, 1998–2005. Journal of Studies on Alcohol and Drugs (Suppl. 16):12–20, 2009.

12. Hingson, R.; Heeren, T.; Winter, M.; et al. Magnitude of alcohol-related mortality and morbidity among U.S. college students ages 18–24: Changes from 1998 to 2001. Annual Review of Public Health 26:259–279, 2005.

13. Wechsler, H, Dowdall, G.W. Maenner. G et al. Changes in binge drinking and related problems among American college students between 1993 and 1997. Results of the Harvard School of Public Health College Alcohol Study. Journal of American College Health 47(2):57–68, 1998.

14. Wilcox HC, Conner KR, Caine ED. Association of alcohol and drug use disorders and completed suicide: an empirical review of cohort studies. Drug and Alcohol Dependence. 2004;76(Suppl):S11–19.

15. Rehm J, Baliunas D, Borges GL, Graham K, Irving H, Kehoe T, et al. The relation between different dimensions of alcohol consumption and burden of disease: an overview. Addiction. 2010;105(5):817-43.

16. Castaneda R, Sussman N, Westreich L, Levy R, O'Malley M. A review of the effects of moderate alcohol intake on the treatment of anxiety and mood disorders. J Clin Psychiatry 1996;57(5):207–212.

17. Booth BM, Feng W. The impact of drinking and drinking consequences on short-term employment outcomes in at-risk drinkers in six southern states. J Behavioral Health Services and Research 2002;29(2):157–166.

18. Leonard KE, Rothbard JC. Alcohol and the marriage effect. J Stud Alcohol Suppl 1999;13:139–146.

19. Crews FT. Alcohol-Related Neurodegeneration and Recovery: Mechanisms from Animal Models. Alcohol Research & Health. 2008;31(4):377-388.

20. Yoon, Y.H., and Chen, C.M. Surveillance Report #105: Liver Cirrhosis Mortality in the United States: National, State, and Regional Trends, 2000–2013. Bethesda, MD: National Institute on Alcohol Abuse and Alcoholism (NIAAA), 2016.

21. Singal, A.K.; Guturu, P.; Hmoud, B.; et al. Evolving frequency and outcomes of liver transplantation based on etiology of liver disease. Transplantation 95(5):755–760, 2013. PMID: 23370710.

22. National Cancer Institute. Alcohol Consumption, November 2015 update. Available at: http://www.progressreport.cancer.gov/prevention/alcohol. Accessed 9/19/16.

23. World Health Organization (WHO), Global Health Observatory (GHO) [8/31/2012]; Available at: http://www.who.int/gho/substance_abuse/en/index.html.
24. Read JP, Kahler CW, Stevenson JF. Bridging the gap between alcoholism treatment and practice: What works and why. Professional Psychology: Research and Practice. 2001;32:227–238.
25. New Alcohol Use Disorder Guideline Emphasizes Medication - Medscape - Jan 10, 2018.
26. Miller WR, Walters ST, Bennett ME. How effective is alcoholism treatment in the United States? J Stud Alcohol. 2001;62:211–20.
27. Brown RA, Abrantes AM, Read JP, et al. Aerobic Exercise for Alcohol Recovery: Rationale, Program Description, and Preliminary Findings. Behavior modification. 2009;33(2):220-249. doi:10.1177/0145445508329112.
28. Zgierska A, Rabago D, Zuelsdorff M, Coe C, Miller M, Fleming M. Mindfulness Meditation for Alcohol Relapse Prevention: A Feasibility Pilot Study. Journal of addiction medicine. 2008;2(3):165-173. doi:10.1097/ADM.0b013e31816f8546.
29. Behere RV, Muralidharan K, Benegal V. Complementary and alternative medicine in the treatment of substance use disorders--a review of the evidence. Drug Alcohol Rev. 2009 May;28(3):292-300.
30. Hallgren M, Romberg K, Bakshi AS and ANdreasson S. Yoga as an adjunct treatment for alcohol dependence: a pilot study. Complement Ther Med. 2014 Jun;22(3):441-5. doi: 10.1016/j.ctim.2014.03.003. Epub 2014 Mar 15.
31. Khalsa SBS, Khalsa GS, Khalsa HK, Khalsa MK. Evaluation of a residential Kundalini yoga lifestyle pilot program for addiction in India. J Ethn Subst Abuse 2008;7:67–79.
32. Vedamurthachar A, Janakiramaiah N, Hegde JM, et al. Antidepressant efficacy and hormonal effects of Sudarshana Kriya Yoga (SKY) in alcohol dependent individuals. J Affect Disord 2006;94:249–253.
33. Badrick E, Bobak M, Britton A, Kirschbaum C, Marmot M, Kumari M. The Relationship between Alcohol Consumption and Cortisol Secretion in an Aging Cohort. The Journal of Clinical Endocrinology and Metabolism. 2008;93(3):750-757. doi:10.1210/jc.2007-0737.
34. A. K. Rose, S. G. Shaw, M. A. Prendergast and H. J. Little. The Importance of Glucocorticoids in Alcohol Dependence and Neurotoxicity. Alcoholism: Clinical & Experimental Research, 7 SEP 2010.
35. Reddy S, Dick AM, Gerber MR, Mitchell K. The Effect of a Yoga Intervention on Alcohol and Drug Abuse Risk in Veteran and Civilian Women with Posttraumatic Stress Disorder. Journal of Alternative and Complementary Medicine. 2014;20(10):750-756. doi:10.1089/acm.2014.0014.
36. Khanna S, Greeson JM. A Narrative Review of Yoga and Mindfulness as Complementary Therapies for Addiction. Complementary therapies in medicine. 2013;21(3):244-252. doi:10.1016/j.ctim.2013.01.008.

37. Shafil M. Lavely R, Jaffe R. Meditation and the prevention of alcohol abuse. Am J Psychiatry. 1975 Sep;132(9):942-5.
38. Monahan RJ. Secondary prevention of drug dependence through the transcendental meditation program in metropolitan Philadelphia. Int. J Addict. 1977 Sep;12(6):729-54.
39. Garland EL, Gaylord SA, Boettiger CA, Howard MO. Mindfulness training modifies cognitive, affective, and physiological mechanisms implicated in alcohol dependence: results of a randomized controlled pilot trial. J Psychoactive Drugs. 2010;42(2):177–92.
40. Schroder KE, Perrine MW. Covariations of emotional states and alcohol consumption: evidence from 2 years of daily data collection. Soc Sci Med. 2007;65(12):2588–2602.
41. Sinha R. The role of stress in addiction relapse. Current Psychiatry Reports. 2007;9(5):388–395.
42. Chong, Cecilia SM, Tsunaka et al. Effects of Yoga on Stress Management in Healthy Adults: A Systematic Review. Alternative Therapies in Health and Medicine, Vol. 17, Iss.i, Jan/Feb 2011: 32-8.
43. Goyal M, Singh S, Sibinga EMS, et al. Meditation Programs for Psychological Stress and Well-being: A Systematic Review and Meta-analysis. JAMA internal medicine. 2014;174(3):357-368. doi:10.1001/jamainternmed.2013.13018.

Alzheimer's Disease

Alzheimer's disease (AD), the most common form of dementia, is a complex disease characterized by an accumulation of β-amyloid plaques and neurofibrillary tangles composed of tau amyloid fibrils[1], and this is associated with synapse loss and neurodegeneration. The result is memory impairment and other cognitive problems. There is currently no known treatment that slows the progression of this disorder. In the US, approximately 5.5 million people are affected. It is the sixth leading cause of death in the US[2]. According to the 2014 World Alzheimer report, the prevalence worldwide is estimated to be as high 44 million people, and its prevalence is expected to triple by 2050. Recent evidence indicates that changes in olfaction, hearing, and even walking speed may precede the onset of cognitive impairments and dementia by 5–15 years, and are strong risk factors for AD dementia[3,4]. Substantial evidence exists to indicate that the pathophysiologic processes of AD, in these patients, are present in the brain, well in advance of subjective or objective deficits[5]. Risk factors include hypertension[6], diabetes mellitus[7], low or high body weight[8-9], smoking[10], traumatic brain injury[11] and a diet high in fat, especially trans-unsaturated fats[12-13]. Diagnosis is mainly based on clinical symptoms. There is no specific diagnostic test. Brain imaging is sometimes performed, primarily to rule out other causes of dementia, like tumors. Several biomarkers of this diseases are being evaluated. Pharmacologic treatment is based on the use of cholinesterase inhibitors and memantine, sometimes used concomitantly. Creating a safe environment, proper diet and exercise are all helpful for these patients.

Yoga and Alzheimer's Disease

There are no direct studies of yoga practice in Alzheimer's disease patients, However, many investigations in other neurological diseases have suggested that yoga should help these patients[14]. Yoga reduces stress[15] and stress damages hippocampal cells[16]. Stress results in memory and cognitive decline[17-18] and reduction of stress with meditation[19] may help AD patients. Cortisol levels are higher in AD patients[20] and increase as the disease progresses, while they do not increase in non-AD patients that were also aging[21]. Some yoga modalities, especially meditation, help reduce cortisol levels[22].

Family members usually become the caregivers of Alzheimer's disease patients[23], and are subjected to a significant physical and mental burden[24]. In a study of 46 AD patient family caregivers, participants were randomly assigned (for 2-months) to a stress-reduction program, with 25 in the yoga and compassion meditation group and 25 in an untreated control group. At the end of the study, there was a greater reduction in stress, anxiety and depression in the yoga group. The yoga group also demonstrated a reduction in the concentration of salivary cortisol[25].

Another study demonstrated that brief daily meditation practices by family dementia caregivers decreased their depression and improved mental and cognitive functioning[26].

Conclusion

Yoga may help patients and caregivers with Alzheimer's disease – but more research is needed.

References

1. Hardy J. Alzheimer's disease: the amyloid cascade hypothesis: an update and reappraisal. J Alzheimers Dis. 2006;9(Suppl 3):151–153.
2. alz.org/facts/
3. Devanand DP, Liu X, Tabert MH, Pradhaban G, Cuasay K, Bell K, et al. Combining early markers strongly predicts conversion from mild cognitive impairment to Alzheimer's disease. Biol Psychiatry. 2008;64(10):871–9.
4. Albers MW, Gilmore GC, Kaye J, et al. At the interface of sensory and motor dysfunctions and Alzheimer's Disease. Alzheimer's & dementia□: The Journal of the Alzheimer's Association. 2015;11(1):70-98. doi:10.1016/j.jalz.2014.04.514.
5. Sperling RA, Aisen PS, Beckett LA, Bennett DA, Craft S, Fagan AM, et al. Toward defining the preclinical stages of Alzheimer's disease: Recommendations from the National Institute on Aging-Alzheimer's Association workgroups on diagnostic guidelines for Alzheimer's disease. Alzheimers Dement. 2011;7:280–92.
6. Whitmer RA, Sidney S, Selby J, Johnston SC, Yaffe K 2005b. Midlife cardiovascular risk factors and risk of dementia in late life. Neurology 64: 277–281.
7. Profenno LA, Porsteinsson AP, Faraone SV 2009. Meta-analysis of Alzheimer's disease risk with obesity, diabetes, and related disorders. Biol Psychiat 67: 505–512.

8. Faxen-Irving G, Basun H, Cederholm T 2005. Nutritional and cognitive relationships and long-term mortality in patients with various dementia disorders. Age Ageing 34: 136–141.
9. Profenno LA, Porsteinsson AP, Faraone SV 2009. Meta-analysis of Alzheimer's disease risk with obesity, diabetes, and related disorders. Biol Psychiat 67: 505–512.
10. Whitehouse PJ, Martino AM, Wagster MV, Price DL, Mayeux R, Atack JR, Kellar KJ 1988. Reductions in [3H] nicotinic acetylcholine binding in Alzheimer's disease and Parkinson's disease: An autoradiographic study. Neurology 38: 720–723.
11. Fleminger S, Oliver DL, Lovestone S, Rabe-Hesketh S, Giora A 2003. Head injury as a risk factor for Alzheimer's disease: The evidence 10 years on; a partial replication. J Neurol Neurosurg Psychiat 74: 857–862.
12. Luchsinger JA, Tang MX, Shea S, Mayeux R 2002. Caloric intake and the risk of Alzheimer disease. Arch Neurol 59: 1258–1263.
13. Morris MC, Evans DA, Bienias JL, Tangney CC, Bennett DA, Aggarwal N, Schneider J, Wilson RS 2003. Dietary fats and the risk of incident Alzheimer disease. Arch Neurol 60: 194–200.
14. Mishra SK, Singh P, Bunch SJ, Zhang R. The therapeutic value of yoga in neurological disorders. Annals of Indian Academy of Neurology. 2012;15(4):247-254. doi:10.4103/0972-2327.104328.
15. Chong CS, Tsunaka M, Tsang HW, Chan EP, Cheung WM. Effects of yoga on stress management in healthy adults: a systematic review. Alternative Therapies in Health and Medicine. 2011;17(1):32–38.
16. Lupien SJ, de Leon M, de Santi S, Convit A, Tarshish C, Nair NPV, et al. Cortisol levels during human aging predict hippocampal atrophy and memory deficits. Nature Neuroscience. 1998;1:69–73.
17. Kabat-Zinn J, Massion AO, Kristeller J, Peterson LG, Fletcher KE, Pbert L, et al. Effectiveness of a meditation-based stress reduction program in the treatment of anxiety disorders. Am J Psychiatry. 1992;149:936–43.
18. Carlson LE, Ursuliak Z, Goodey E, Angen M, Speca M. The effects of a mindfulness meditation-based stress reduction program on mood and symptoms of stress in cancer outpatients: 6-month follow-up. Support Care Cancer. 2001;9:112–23.
19. Marchand W. R. Mindfulness-based stress reduction, mindfulness-based cognitive therapy, and Zen meditation for depression, anxiety, pain, and psychological distress. J Psychiatr Pract 18, 233–252 (2012).
20. Davis KL, Davis BM, Greenwald BS, Mohs RC, Mathe AA, Johns CA, et al. Cortisol and Alzheimer's disease, I: Basal studies. Am J Psychiatry. 1986;143:300–5.
21. Weiner MF, Vobach S, Olsson K, Svetlik D, Risser RC. Cortisol Secretion and Alzheimer's Disease Progression. Biol Psychiatry. 1997;42:1030–8.
22. Raghavendra RM, Vadiraja HS, Nagarathna R, Nagendra HR, Rekha M, Vanitha N, et al. Effects of a Yoga Program on Cortisol Rhythm and Mood States in Early Breast Cancer Patients Undergoing Adjuvant Radiotherapy: A Randomized Controlled Trial. Integr Cancer Ther. 2009;8:37–46.
23. R. Stone, G. L. Cafferata, and J. Sangl, "Caregivers of the frail elderly: a national profile," Gerontologist, vol. 27, no. 5, pp. 616–626, 1987.

24. R. Schulz and S. R. Beach, "Caregiving as a risk factor for mortality: the caregiver health effects study," Journal of the American Medical Association, vol. 282, no. 23, pp. 2215–2219, 1999.
25. M. A. D. Danucalov, E. H. Kozasa, K. T. Ribas, J. C. F. Galduróz, M. C. Garcia, I. T. N. Verreschi, K. C. Oliveira, L. Romani de Oliveira, J. R. Leite. A Yoga and Compassion Meditation Program Reduces Stress in Familial Caregivers of Alzheimer's Disease Patients. Evid Based Complement Alternat Med. 2013; 2013: 513149. Published online 2013 Apr 18.
26. Lavretsky H, Siddarth P, Nazarian N, et al. A pilot study of yogic meditation for family dementia caregivers with depressive symptoms: Effects on mental health, cognition, and telomerase activity. International journal of geriatric psychiatry. 2013;28(1):57-65. doi:10.1002/gps.3790.

Anxiety

According to the Anxiety and Depression Association of America, anxiety disorders affect over 40 million adults in the United States (age 18 and older), or 18.1% of the population every year[1]. The major anxiety disorders include generalized anxiety disorder (GAD), panic disorder (PD) and social anxiety disorder (SAD). GAD is twice as common in women, when compared to men. It affects 6.8 million adults, or 3.1% of the U.S. population. PD affects 6 million adults, or 2.7% of the U.S. population. Like GAD, it is twice as common in women. SAD affects 15 million adults, or 6.8% of the U.S. population. It is seen equally among women and men. Anxiety disorders represent the most common mental illness in the U.S. Phobias and separation anxiety disorders are also included in the anxiety disorders group. It is estimated that 7%-9% of the population suffers from specific phobias while 1%-2% of the US population exhibits pathological separation anxiety[2]. Anxiety often accompanies depression and is also a facet of panic attacks, post-traumatic stress disorder (PTSD) and obsessive-compulsive disorder (OCD). Lifetime prevalence of anxiety disorders is as high as 31%[3].

In general, anxiety disorders are characterized by emotions of apprehension or dread, restlessness or irritability, catastrophizing and feeling tense. These feelings may be associated with a racing heart, shortness of breath, sweating, tremors, fatigue and GI symptoms such as diarrhea.

Anxiety disorders are treated with pharmacotherapy and/or psychotherapy[4]. Drugs commonly used include fluoxetine, paroxetine, citalopram, escitalopram, sertraline, and mirtazapine. Benzodiazepines are sometimes used for intravenous or oral acute sedation. Many other drugs may also be used, depending upon the specificity and severity of the anxiety disorder. In addition, cognitive and behavioral psychotherapy is also used, alone or in combination with pharmacotherapy. Unfortunately, anxiety disorders are often under-diagnosed[5] and many remain under-treated[6]. Anxiolytic drugs have side effects[7] and patients are often not motivated to take psychotherapy[8].

Yoga and Anxiety

The therapeutic value of yoga in anxiety disorders has been well studied[9-10]. Kirkwood and associates[11] reviewed eight studies in 2005. They reported that yoga was associated with a positive response in patients suffering from OCD[12], examination anxiety[12-14], snake phobia[15], anxiety neurosis[16], and psychoneurosis[17.] Anxiety neurosis and psychoneurosis are terms no longer used.

Asana practice helps in reducing extreme stress. In a study by Michalsen and associates[18], 24 self-referred emotionally distressed female subjects (mean age 37.9+/-7.3 years) who perceived themselves as emotionally distressed, participated in a yoga study. Some women were enrolled in a yoga course, while others were placed on the waiting list. The yoga group attended two-weekly 90-min Iyengar yoga classes. Objective testing was done on entry and after 3 months by Cohen Perceived Stress Scale, State-Trait Anxiety Inventory, Profile of Mood States, CESD-Depression Scale, Bf-S/Bf-S' Well-Being Scales, Freiburg Complaint List and ratings of physical well-being. Compared to waiting-list, the women in the yoga-training demonstrated pronounced and significant improvements in perceived stress, State and Trait Anxiety, well-being, vigor, fatigue and depression. Salivary cortisol decreased significantly after participation in a yoga class.

Breathing exercises have shown to reduce test anxiety. One study[19] involved 107 students who were randomly assigned to control and experimental groups. The students of the experimental group practiced simple pranayama for one full semester. Both groups were tested with the Sarason's test anxiety scale in the final session, before taking the academic examination. In this study, only 33.3% of the pranayama practitioners revealed high test anxiety, while 66.7% of the participants in the control group had high test anxiety. Sudharshin Kriya yoga breathing has also shown to reduce anxiety in patients[20].

Meditation is a major part of yoga practice. Meditation has an anxiety reducing effect[21]. In a meta-analysis of studies on transcendental meditation and reduction in anxiety, the positive effect in anxiety reduction was more in patients with the highest level of anxiety at the outset[22].

In patients with drug resistant anxiety, mindfulness meditation has showed significant reduction. Using the Beck Anxiety Inventory, Tang and associates[23] found significant reduction in anxiety scores in patients with epilepsy with yoga intervention. The benefit was confirmed by a significant reduction in anxiety in the intervention group using McNemar tests.

Yoga practice has shown to reduce anxiety in a diverse group of people. These include medical students[24], young musicians[25], police academy trainees[26], military personnel with PTSD[27], second and third grade students[28], adolescents with learning difficulties[29], and urban youth[30].

Overall, studies of yoga in anxiety states suggest a positive response[31-32]. Yoga participation in patients with anxiety disorders is generally free of any adverse effects[33]. However, low participation and a high attrition rate is often seen.[34-36].

Conclusion

Yoga is beneficial in patients suffering from anxiety disorders and can be used along with pharmacotherapy and psychotherapy.

References

1. adaa.org – accessed 12/31/17.
2. psychiatry.org/patients-families/anxiety-disorders/what-are-anxiety-disorders - accessed 12/31/17.
3. Kessler RC, Angermeyer M, Anthony JC, R DG, Demyttenaere K, Gasquet I, G DG, Gluzman S, Gureje O, Haro JM. et al. Lifetime prevalence and age-of-onset distributions of mental disorders in the World Health Organization's World Mental Health Survey Initiative. World Psychiatry. 2007;6:168–176.
4. de Beurs E; van Balkom AJ; Van Dyck R; Lange A. Long-term outcome of pharmacological and psychological treatment for panic disorder with agoraphobia: a 2-year naturalistic follow-up. Acta Psychiatr Scand. 1999; 99(1):59-67.
5. Vermani M, Marcus M, Katzman MA. Rates of detection of mood and anxiety disorders in primary care: a descriptive, cross-sectional study. Prim Care Companion CNS Disord. 2011;13 doi 10.4088/PCC.4010m01013.

6. Weisberg RB, Dyck I, Culpepper L, Keller MB. Psychiatric Treatment in Primary Care Patients with Anxiety Disorders: A Comparison of Care Received from Primary Care Providers and Psychiatrists. The American journal of psychiatry. 2007;164(2):10.1176/appi.ajp.164.2.276.
7. Practice guideline for the treatment of patients with panic disorder. psychiatryonline.org/content.aspx?bookid=28&sectionid=1680635.
8. Combs H, Markman J. Anxiety disorders in primary care. Med Clin North Am. 2014;98:1007–1023. doi: 10.1016/j.mcna.2014.06.003.
9. Saeed SA, Antonacci DJ, Bloch RM. Exercise, yoga, and meditation for depressive and anxiety disorders. American Family Physician. 2010;81(8):981–987.
10. Hofmann SG, Andreoli G, Carpenter JK, Curtiss J. Effect of Hatha Yoga on Anxiety: A Meta-Analysis. Journal of evidence-based medicine. May 2016:10.1111/jebm.12204. doi:10.1111/jebm.12204.
11. Kirkwood G, Rampes H, Tuffrey V, Richardson J, Pilkington K, Ramaratnam S. Yoga for anxiety: a systematic review of the research evidence. British Journal of Sports Medicine. 2005;39(12):884-891. doi:10.1136/bjsm.2005.018069.
12. Shannahoff-Khalsa DS, Ray LE, Levine S, et al. Randomized controlled trial of yogic meditation techniques for patients with obsessive-compulsive disorder. CNS Spectr 1999;4:34–47.
13. Broota A, Sanghvi C. Efficacy of two relaxation techniques in examination anxiety. Journal of Personality Clinical Studies1994;10:29–35.
14. Malathi A, Damodaran A. Stress due to exams in medical students: role of yoga. Indian J Physiol Pharmacol1999;43:218–24.
15. Norton GR, Johnson WE. A comparison of two relaxation procedures for reducing cognitive and somatic anxiety. J Behav Ther Exp Psychiatry1983;14:209–14.
16. Sharma I, Azmi SA, Settiwar RM. Evaluation of the effect of pranayama in anxiety state. Alternative Medicine1991;3:227–35.
17. Vahia NS, Doongaji DR, Jeste DV, et al. Psychophysiologic therapy based on the concepts of Patanjali. A new approach to the treatment of neurotic and psychosomatic disorders. Am J Psychother 1973;27:557–65.
18. Michalsen A, Grossman P, Acil A, Langhorst J, Ludtke R, Esch T, et al. Rapid stress reduction and anxiolysis among distressed women because of a three-month intensive yoga program. Med Sci Monit (2005) 11(12):CR555–61.
19. Nemati A. The effect of pranayama on test anxiety and test performance. International Journal of Yoga. 2013;6(1):55-60. doi:10.4103/0973-6131.105947.
20. Brown RP, Gerbarg PL. Sudarshan Kriya Yogic breathing in the treatment of stress, anxiety, and depression: part II—clinical applications and guidelines. Journal of Alternative and Complementary Medicine. 2005;11(4):711–717.
21. Chen KW, Berger CC, Manheimer E, Forde D, Magidson J, Dachman L, Lejuez CW. Meditative therapies for reducing anxiety: a systematic

review and meta-analysis of randomized controlled trials. Depress Anxiety. 2012 Jul;29(7):545-62. doi: 10.1002/da.21964. Epub 2012 Jun 14.

22. Orme-Johnson DW, Barnes VA. Effects of the transcendental meditation technique on trait anxiety: a meta-analysis of randomized controlled trials. J Altern Complement Med (2003) 19:1–12.10.1089/acm.2013.0204.

23. Tang V, Poon WS, Kwan P. Mindfulness-based therapy for drug-resistant epilepsy: an assessor-blinded randomized trial. Neurology. 2015;85(13):1100–7.

24. Malathi A, Damodaran A. Stress due to exams in medical students – Role of yoga. Indian J Physiol Pharmacol. 1999;43:218–24.

25. Khalsa SB, Shorter SM, Cope S, Wyshak G, Sklar E. Yoga ameliorates performance anxiety and mood disturbance in young professional musicians. Appl Psychophysiol Biofeedback. 2009 Dec;34(4):279-89. doi: 10.1007/s10484-009-9103-4. Epub 2009 Aug 6.

26. Jeter PE, Cronin S, Khalsa SB. Evaluation of the benefits of a kripalu yoga program for police academy trainees: a pilot study. Int J Yoga Therap. 2013;23(1):24-30.

27. Johnston JM, Minami T, Greenwald D, et al. Yoga for military service personnel with PTSD: A single arm study. Psychol Trauma. 2015 Nov;7(6):555-62. doi: 10.1037/tra0000051. Epub 2015 May 25.

28. Butzer B., Day D., Potts A., et al. Effects of a classroom-based yoga intervention on cortisol and behavior in second- and third-grade students: A pilot study. Journal of Evidence-Based Complementary and Alternative Medicine. 2015;20(1):41–49.

29. Beauchemin J., Hutchins T. L., Patterson F. Mindfulness meditation may lessen anxiety, promote social skills, and improve academic performance among adolescents with learning disabilities. Complementary Health Practice Review. 2008;13(1):34–45.

30. Sibinga E. M. S., Kerrigan D., Stewart M., Johnson K., Magyari T., Ellen J. M. Mindfulness-based stress reduction for urban youth. The Journal of Alternative and Complementary Medicine. 2011;17(3):213–218.

31. Khalsa MK, Greiner-Ferris JM, Hofmann SG, Khalsa SBS. Yoga-Enhanced Cognitive Behavioral Therapy (Y-CBT) for Anxiety Management: A Pilot Study. Clinical psychology & psychotherapy. 2015;22(4):364-371. doi:10.1002/cpp.1902.

32. Duan-Porter W, Coeytaux RR, McDuffie J, et al. Evidence Map of Yoga for Depression, Anxiety, and Posttraumatic Stress Disorder. Journal of physical activity & health. 2016;13(3):281-288. doi:10.1123/jpah.2015-0027.

33. Shannahoff-Khalsa DS, Ray LE, Levine S, et al. Randomized controlled trial of yogic meditation techniques for patients with obsessive-compulsive disorder. CNS Spectr 1999;4:34–47.

34. Shannahoff-Khalsa DS, Ray LE, Levine S, et al. Randomized controlled trial of yogic meditation techniques for patients with obsessive-compulsive disorder. CNS Spectr 1999;4:34–47.

35. Sahasi G, Mohan D, Kacker C. Effectiveness of yogic techniques in the management of anxiety. Journal of Personality Clinical Studies1989;5:51–5.
36. Sharma I, Azmi SA, Settiwar RM. Evaluation of the effect of pranayama in anxiety state. Alternative Medicine1991;3:227–35.

Asthma

About 300 million people have asthma globally[1-3]. It is a common disease among children[4] and most asthma-related deaths occur in low and lower-middle income countries[5]. Asthma is characterized by reversible airway obstruction. It is characterized by wheezing – a musical high-pitched whistling sound, initially present at the end of expiration and with an increase in severity of the disease, throughout the expiration or also during inspiration. If asthma involves the lower airways, wheezing may not be evident. In exercise-induced or nocturnal asthma, the only presenting symptom may be cough. The National Asthma Education and Prevention Program recommends that diagnosis be based on symptoms of episodic airflow obstruction with symptoms being at least partially reversible. No other cause explaining the symptoms should be present[6]. Patients with asthma may show blood eosinophilia greater than 4% or >300-400/μL. Pulse oximetry in children may provide an estimate of the degree of asthma: 97% or above is mild asthma, 92-97% is moderate asthma, and less than 92% signifies severe asthma. Asthmatics will demonstrate a reduced ratio of forced expiratory volume in 1st sec (FEV1) to forced vital capacity, when compared with predicted values and show an increase of 12% and 200 mL after the administration of a short-acting bronchodilator. Bronchoprovocation with methacholine is sometimes used to demonstrate bronchial hyperreactivity. Many other tests like chest x-ray, MRI and arterial blood gasses may be used to assist in the diagnosis.

Treatment includes agents to control asthmatic attacks such as inhaled corticosteroids, long-acting bronchodilators (beta-agonists and anticholinergics), theophylline, leukotriene modifiers, anti-immunoglobulin E antibodies and anti-IL-5 antibodies. Treatment is also directed at relief from attacks, and these medications include short-acting bronchodilators, systemic corticosteroids, and ipratropium. Complementary and alternative medicine is also used by patients with asthma[7]. This includes yoga[8].

Yoga and Asthma

Several studies have shown an improvement in the pulmonary function parameters of asthmatic patients with yoga practice[9]. In one study, sixty stable asthma patients were randomized into a yoga group (yoga intervention for 2 months) and a control group. The former group demonstrated a significant improvement in forced vital capacity, forced expiratory volume in 1st sec, peak expiratory flow rate, maximum voluntary ventilation and slow vital capacity when compared to the control group[10].

Asthma is characterized by bronchial inflammation[11]. Improvement in inflammation was noted in a study of 276 patients with mild to moderate asthma (FEV 1> 60%), aged between 12 to 60 years. The randomly assigned yoga group received yogic intervention in addition to medical treatment while the control group received only standard medical treatment. Biochemical assessment was carried out at baseline and after 6 months of the study. The yoga group demonstrated significant decrease in total leukocyte count and differential leukocytes count in comparison to control group[12].

In a study of 24 asthma patients randomized into a yoga group and control group, yoga exercises in the former (50 minutes a day for 4 weeks) resulted in a decreased number asthma attacks. The medication uses also decreased. These patients also showed a significant improvement in the peak expiratory flow rate[13]. A decrease in the frequency of medication use has been noted before in asthma patients with the practice of yoga[14].

Asthmatics suffer from associated anxiety and stress, and these emotional factors are positively impacted by yoga[15-17]. Several studies have demonstrated that yoga also improves the quality of life in patients with asthma[18-20].

In a systemic review and meta-analysis of fourteen randomized controlled trials with 824 patients, Cramer and associates confirmed the improvements noted in asthma patient with the practice of yoga. They suggested that yoga "be considered an ancillary intervention or an alternative to breathing exercises for asthma patients interested in complementary interventions"[21]. No adverse effects were noted.

Conclusion

Yoga is emerging as a valuable complementary therapeutic modality in bronchial asthma.

References

1. Masoli M, Fabian D, Holt S, Beasley R. Global Initiative for Asthma (GINA) Program. The global burden of asthma: Executive summary of the GINA Dissemination Committee report. Allergy. 2004;59: 469–78.
2. Bateman ED, Jithoo A. Asthma and allergy-A global perspective. Allergy. 2007; 62:213–5.
3. Beasley R. The Global Burden of Asthma Report. Global Initiative for Asthma (GINA) 2011. Available from: ginaasthma.org- accessed 12/28/17.
4. cdc.gov/nchs/products/hestats.htm- accessed 12/28/17.
5. WHO: http://www.who.int/mediacentre/factsheets/fs307/en/ - accessed 6 October 2015.
6. nhlbi.nih.gov/files/docs/guidelines/asthgdln.pdf - accessed 12/30/17.
7. Slader CA, Reddel HK, Jenkins CR, Armour CL, Bosnic-Anticevich SZ. Complementary and alternative medicine use in asthma: who is using what? Respirology. 2006 Jul;11(4):373-87.
8. Vempati R, Bijlani RL, Deepak KK. The efficacy of a comprehensive lifestyle modification programme based on yoga in the management of bronchial asthma: A randomized controlled trial. BMC Pulm Med.2009; 9:37.
9. Sathyaprabha TN, Murthy H, Murthy BT. Efficacy of naturopathy and yoga in bronchial asthma -- a self controlled matched scientific study. Indian J Physiol Pharmacol. 2001 Jan;45(1):80-6.
10. Singh S, Soni R, Singh KP, Tandon OP. Effect of yoga practices on pulmonary function tests including transfer factor of lung for carbon monoxide (TLCO) in asthma patients. Indian J Physiol Pharmacol. 2012 Jan-Mar;56(1):63-8.
11. Bentley AM, Menz G, Storz C, Robinson DS, et al. Identification of T lymphocytes, macrophages, and activated eosinophils in the bronchial mucosa in intrinsic asthma. Relationship to symptoms and bronchial responsiveness. Am Rev Respir Dis. 1992 Aug;146(2):500-6.
12. Agnihotri S, Kant S, Kumar S, Mishra RK, Mishra SK. Impact of yoga on biochemical profile of asthmatics: A randomized controlled study. International Journal of Yoga. 2014;7(1):17-21. doi:10.4103/0973-6131.123473.
13. Demeke Mekonnen, Andualem Mossie. Clinical Effects of Yoga on Asthmatic Patients: A Preliminary Clinical Trial. Ethiop J Health Sci. 2010 Jul; 20(2): 107–112.
14. Vempati R, Bijlani RL, Deepak KK. The efficacy of a comprehensive lifestyle modification programme based on yoga in the management of bronchial asthma: A randomized controlled trial. BMC Pulm Med.2009; 9:37.
15. Platania-Solazzo A, Field TM, Blank J, et al. Relaxation therapy reduces anxiety in child and adolescent psychiatric patients. Acta Paedopsychiatr. 1992;55(2):115–120.
16. Stuck M, Gloeckner N. Yoga for children in the mirror of the science: working spectrum and practice fields of the training of relaxation with

elements of yoga for children. Early Child Develop Care. 2005;175(4):371–377.

17. West J, Otte C, Geher K, et al. Effects of Hatha yoga and African dance on perceived stress, affect, and salivary cortisol. Ann Behav Med. 2004;28(2):114–118.

18. Vempati R, Bijlani RL, Deepak KK. The efficacy of a comprehensive lifestyle modification programme based on yoga in the management of bronchial asthma: A randomized controlled trial. BMC Pulm Med.2009; 9:37.

19. Bidwell AJ, Yazel B, Davin D, et al. Yoga training improves quality of life in women with asthma. J Altern Complement Med. 2012 Aug;18(8):749-55.

20. Sodhi C, Singh S, Bery A. Assessment of the quality of life in patients with bronchial asthma, before and after yoga: a randomised trial. Iran J Allergy Asthma Immunol. 2014 Feb;13(1): 55-60.

21. Cramer H, Posadzki P, Dobos G, et al. Yoga for asthma: a systematic review and meta-analysis. Ann Allergy Asthma Immunol. 2014 Jun;112(6):503-510.

Attention deficit Hyperactivity Disorder (ADHD)

Attention deficit/hyperactivity disorder (ADHD) is the most common neurobehavioral developmental disorder among school-age children. It is widespread, chronic and often debilitating. According to the American Psychiatric Association's DSM-V, a child diagnosed with ADHD must have symptoms before the age of 12, for at least six months, and affecting two domains of life – inattention and hyperactivity. ADHD is split into three subtypes: primarily inattentive (20–30% of diagnosed population), primarily hyperactive-impulsive (less than 15%), and combined subtype (50–75%)[1]. It is associated with poor academic performance[2], difficulty in socializing[3], and strained family relationships[4]. It often continues into the adult life and may be associated with depression, mood disorders and substance abuse – disrupting the individual's personal and professional life.

According to the Centers for Disease Control and Prevention, data reported in 2011-2012 indicates that approximately 11% of children 4-17 years of age (6.4 million) have been diagnosed with ADHD in the USA [5]. Boys are more likely to have ADHD, with the incidence being 12.1% in boys and 5.5% in girls. ADHD is also prevalent worldwide, affecting 8%-12% of the global children population[6]. ADHD symptoms often continue throughout life[7].

The standard treatment is stimulant medications - such as methylphenidate and amphetamine[8]. Non-stimulant medications such as atomoxetine, clonidine or guanfacine, are also used. It is estimated that in the USA, 69% of children with current ADHD or a total of approximately 3.5 million children are taking medication for ADHD[9]. The medications available demonstrate good efficacy[10], but side effects such as trouble falling asleep, decreased appetite, headaches, abdominal discomfort, and irritability, are often reported[11]. Behavioral interventions also are used therapeutically[12]. Studies reveal that persistence and adherence to pharmacologic treatments for ADHD have been generally inadequate[13].

Yoga and ADHD

Several integrative modalities have also been tried for this disorder[14]. Yoga therapy has been tried in many patients with ADHD. In a small study of 9 children (8 males, 1 female), after an average of 8 yoga training sessions, a significant improvement in the ADHD symptoms (as assessed on Conners' abbreviated rating scale, ADHD rating scale-IV and clinical global impression severity scales) were noted at the time of discharge[15].

Peck and associates found that yoga, given for 30 minutes twice a week, for three weeks, improved the time on task for 10 students with ADHD in an educational setting[16]. Another study, involving 11 students (with a control group of 8) revealed that the yoga group had a significant improvement on Test of Variables of Attention Response Time Variability, and greater improvements on the CTRS Global Emotional Lability subscale. The students also appeared more relaxed. This study validated the complementary use of yoga in ADHD students who were on medications[17]. In a study of 24 yoga group children, 8-12 years old, when compared to a control group of 25 children, an eight-week yoga program significantly improved sustained attention and discrimination function in the former[18]. Yoga also improves executive functioning in this population[19].

Meditation intervention has also shown benefits in children with ADHD. In one study, the effects of Sahaja yoga meditation were studied in 48 participants with 31 receiving medication, 14 not on any medication, and 3 with treatment status unknown. The program lasted six weeks and included two per week 90-minute clinic sessions. They also performed meditation at home. Several improvements were noted in these children – improved self-esteem, better sleep, less anxiety, less conflicts and better ability to focus at school. Benefits were also noted in their parents – they were happier, felt less stressed and had a better ability to handle their children's behavior[20].

When mindful meditation is combined with other parenting techniques, children with ADHD do better[21]. In a recent study by Crescentini and group, 6 healthy primary school children ages seven to eight years old were trained in mindfulness meditation, over a period of eight weeks. The sessions were three times a week. Teachers reported a reduction of attention and internalizing issues in these ADHD students[22].

Beneficial effects on ADHD in adolescents have also been recorded. In a study by Van de Weijer-Bergsma et al., ten adolescents, 19 parents and seven academic tutors underwent mindfulness training for eight weeks each session being for 1.5-hours. At the end of the program, the adolescents had improvements in attention problems, executive functioning and performance[23].

Mindful meditation is also effective in adults. In one study, 78% of the 8 adolescents and 24 adults undergoing mindfulness meditation reported a significant reduction in their ADHD symptoms. Significant positive effects were also recorded on other objective pre- and post-testing parameters[24].

Many other studies have confirmed the beneficial effects of multi-component yoga in patients with ADHD.

Conclusion

The objective data is clearly supportive of the use of yoga exercises and mindful meditation as a complementary treatment of ADHD, in children, adolescents and adults. Benefits have also been noted in parents and academic tutors. No safety problems have been reported. Participants did not experience any adverse effects in any of the reported studies.

References

1. Spencer T.J., Biederman J., Mick E. Attention-deficit/hyperactivity disorder: Diagnosis, lifespan, comorbidities, and neurobiology. Ambul. Pediatr. 2007;7:73–81. doi: 10.1016/j.ambp.2006.07.006.
2. Faraone SV, Biederman J, Monuteaux MC, et al. A psychometric measure of learning disability predicts educational failure four years later in boys with ADHD. J Atten Disord. 2001;4:220–30.
3. Bagwell CL, Molina BS, Pelham WE, et al. ADHD and problems in peer relations: Predictions from childhood to adolescence. J Am Acad Child Adolesc Psychiatry. 2001;40:1285–92.
4. Johnston C, Mash EJ. Families of children with ADHD: review and recommendations for future research. Clin Child Fam Psychol Rev2001;4:183–207.

6. Faraone SV, Sergeant J, Gillberg C, Biederman J. The worldwide prevalence of ADHD: Is it an American condition? World Psychiatry. 2003;2:104–13.

7. Brown TE. ADHD Comorbidities: Handbook for ADHD Complications in Children and Adults. Washington, DC: American Psychiatric Press; 2009.

8. Rappley MD. Clinical practice. Attention deficit-hyperactivity disorder. N Engl J Med. 2005;352:165–73.

9. https://www.addrc.org/adhd-data-statistics/ (accessed 12/29/17).

10. Pelham WE, Jr, Carlson C, Sams SE, Vallano G, Dixon MJ, Hoza B. Separate and combined effects of methylphenidate and behavior modification on boys with attention deficit-hyperactivity disorder in the classroom. J Consult Clin Psychol. 1993;61:506–15.

11. Greydanus DE. Pharmacologic treatment of attention-deficit hyperactivity disorder. Indian J Pediatr. 2005;72:953–60.

12. Wolraich M., Brown L., Brown R.T., DuPaul G., Earls M., Feldman H.M., Ganiats T.G., Kaplanek B., Meyer B., Perrin J., et al. ADHD: Clinical practice guideline for the diagnosis, evaluation, and treatment of attention-deficit/hyperactivity disorder in children and adolescents. Pediatrics. 2011;128:1007–1022.

13. Gajria K, Lu M, Sikirica V, et al. Adherence, persistence, and medication discontinuation in patients with attention-deficit/hyperactivity disorder – a systematic literature review. Neuropsychiatric Disease and Treatment. 2014;10:1543-1569. doi:10.2147/NDT.S65721.

14. Sadiq AJ. Attention-deficit/hyperactivity disorder and integrative approaches. Pediatr Ann. 2007;36:508–15.; McClafferty H. Complementary, holistic and integrative medicine. Pediatrics Rev. 2011;32:201–203. doi: 10.1542/pir.32-5-201.

15. Hariprasad VR, Arasappa R, Varambally S, Srinath S, Gangadhar BN. Feasibility and efficacy of yoga as an add-on intervention in attention deficit-hyperactivity disorder: An exploratory study. Indian Journal of Psychiatry. 2013;55(Suppl 3) :S379-S384. doi:10.4103/0019-5545.116317.

16. Peck H.L., Kehle T.J., Bray M.A., Theodore L.A. Yoga as an intervention for children with attention problems. Sch. Psychol. Rev. 2005;34:415–424.

17. Jensen P.S., Kenny D.T. The effects of yoga on the attention and behavior of boys with attention-deficit/hyperactivity disorder (ADHD) J. Atten. Disorders. 2004;7:205–216.

18. Chou C., Huang C. Effects of an 8-week yoga program on sustained attention and discrimination in children with attention deficit hyperactivity disorder. PeerJ. 2017 doi: 10.7717/peerj.2883.

19. Gothe N., Potifex M.B., Hillman C., McAuley E. The acute effects of yoga on executive function. J. Phys. Act. Health. 2013;10:488–495. doi: 10.1123/jpah.10.4.488.

20. Harrison L.J., Manocha R., Rubia K. Sahaja yoga meditation as a family treatment programme for children with attention deficits-hyperactivity

disorder. Clin. Child Psychol. Psychiatry. 2004;9:479–497. doi: 10.1177/1359104504046155.

21. Taren A.A., Gianaros P.J., Greco C.M., Lindsay E.K., Fairgrieve A., Brown K.W., Rosen R.K., Ferris J.L., Julson E., Marsland A.L., et al. Mindfulness meditation training and executive control network resting state functional connectivity: A randomized controlled trial. Psychosom. Med. 2017.

22. Crescentini C., Capurso V., Furlan S., Fabbro F. Mindfulness-oriented meditation for primary school children: Effects on attention and psychological well-being. Front. Psychol. 2016;7 doi: 10.3389/fpsyg.2016.00805.

23. Van de Weijer-Bergsma E., Formsma A.R., de Bruin E.I., Bögels S.M. The effectiveness of mindfulness training on behavioral problems and attentional functioning in adolescents with ADHD. J. Child Fam. Stud. 2012;21:775–787. doi: 10.1007/s10826-011-9531-7.

24. Zylowska L., Ackerman D.L., Yang M.H., Futrell J.L., Horton N.L., Hale T.S., Pataki C., Smalley S.L. Mindfulness meditation training in adults and adolescents with ADHD. J. Atten. Disord. 2008;11:737–746. doi: 10.1177/1087054707308502.

Autism Spectrum Disorder (ASD)

Autism spectrum disorder (ASD) affects more than 3 million individuals in the US. It is more common in boys than girls, with estimates that 1 in 42 boys and 1 in 189 girls are diagnosed with autism in the United States[1]. And these numbers are increasing. It occurs in all racial, ethnic, and socioeconomic groups[2]. About 10% of children with autism are also identified with genetic disorders such as Down syndrome, fragile X syndrome, tuberous sclerosis, or other genetic and chromosomal disorders[3]. About 44% of ASD children have average to above average intellectual ability[4]. ASD commonly co-occurs with other developmental, psychiatric, and neurologic disorders, and this association is as high as in 83%[5]. The co-occurrence of one or more psychiatric diagnoses is 10%[6]. There are no medications available for cure. Treatment is directed at improving functionality in these patients. This includes applied behavior analysis. Complementary and alternative medicine is also used by many patients[7-9]. Yoga has also been tried[10].

Yoga and Autism Spectrum Disorder

Integrated movement therapy is a yoga based therapy that addresses six core principles of therapy for patients for ASD, namely structure and continuity, social interaction, language stimulation, self-calming, physical stimulation, and direct self-esteem building. According to Kenny, this program is usually successful and improves functionality in these patients[11]. GABA (neurotransmitter gamma-aminobutyric acid) inhibitory activity is low in patients with ASD[12]. Yoga helps increase GABA brain levels[13].

In 2011, Rosenblatt et al. found no improvement in the Aberrant Behavioral Checklist Irritability subscale in 24 children with autism using a combined yoga, dance and music therapy program[14]. However, in a study in 2012 by Koenig and associates[15], yielded a significant reduction in teacher-rated Aberrant Behavioral Checklist scores in the intervention group (manualized yoga for 16 weeks). The control group attended standard school morning activities.

Conclusion

Yoga therapy may be helpful in patients with autism spectrum disorder.

References

1. tacanow.org/family-resources/latest-autism-statistics-2/. - accessed 1/12/18.
2. cdc.gov/ncbddd/autism/data.html - accessed 1/12/18.
3. Cohen D, Pichard N, Tordjman S, Baumann C, Burglen L, Excoffier E, Lazar G, Mazet P, Pinquier C, Verloes A, Heron D. Specific genetic disorders and autism: Clinical contribution towards their identification. J Autism Dev Disord. 2005; 35(1): 103-116.
4. Christensen DL, Baio J, Braun KV, et al. Prevalence and Characteristics of Autism Spectrum Disorder Among Children Aged 8 Years — Autism and Developmental Disabilities Monitoring Network, 11 Sites, United States, 2012. MMWR Surveill Summ 2016;65(No. SS-3)(No. SS-3):1–23. doi: dx.doi.org/10.15585/mmwr.ss6503a1.
5. Cohen D, Pichard N, Tordjman S, Baumann C, Burglen L, Excoffier E, Lazar G, Mazet P, Pinquier C, Verloes A, Heron D. Specific genetic disorders and autism: Clinical contribution towards their identification. J Autism Dev Disord. 2005; 35(1): 103-116.
6. Levy SE, Giarelli E, Lee LC, Schieve LA, Kirby RS, Cunniff C, Nicholas J, Reaven J, Rice CE. Autism spectrum disorder and co-occurring developmental, psychiatric, and medical conditions among children in multiple populations of the United States. J Dev Behav Pediatr. 2010 May;31(4):267-75. doi: 10.1097/DBP.0b013e3181d5d03b.
7. Levy, S. Complementary and Alternative Medicine Among Children Recently Diagnosed with Autistic Spectrum Disorder; Journal of Developmental and Behavioral Pediatrics, December 2003; vol 24: pp 418-423.
8. Brondino N, Fusar-Poli L, Rocchetti M, Provenzani U, Barale F, Politi P. Complementary and Alternative Therapies for Autism Spectrum Disorder. Evidence-based Complementary and Alternative Medicine: eCAM. 2015;2015:258589. doi:10.1155/2015/258589.
9. Chan A. S., Sze S. L., Siu N. Y., Lau E. M., Cheung M.-C. A chinese mind-body exercise improves self-control of children with autism: a randomized controlled trial. PLoS ONE. 2013;8(7) doi: 10.1371/journal.pone.0068184.e68184.
10. Kenny M. Integrated movement therapy: yoga-based therapy as a viable and effective intervention for autism spectrum and related disorders. Intern J Yoga Therap 2002;12:71–79.
11. Kenny M. Integrated movement therapy: yoga-based therapy as a viable and effective intervention for autism spectrum and related disorders. Intern J Yoga Therap 2002;12:71–79.

12. Caroline E. Robertson, Eva-Maria Ratai, Nancy Kanwisher. Reduced GABAergic Action in the Autistic Brain. Current Biology. Volume 26, Issue 1, p80–85, 11 January 2016.
13. Streeter C. C., Jensen J. E., Perlmutter R. M., et al. Yoga Asana sessions increase brain GABA levels: a pilot study. Journal of Alternative and Complementary Medicine. 2007;13(4):419–426. doi: 10.1089/acm.2007.6338.
14. Rosenblatt L. E., Gorantla S., Torres J. A., et al. Relaxation response-based yoga improves functioning in young children with autism: a Pilot Study. Journal of Alternative and Complementary Medicine. 2011;17(11):1029–1035. doi: 10.1089/acm.2010.0834.
15. Koenig K. P., Buckley-Reen A., Garg S. Efficacy of the get ready to learn yoga program among children with autism spectrum disorders: a pretest-posttest control group design. American Journal of Occupational Therapy. 2012;66(5):538–546. doi: 10.5014/ajot.2012.004390.

Back Pain

Chronic low back pain is defined as low back pain of at least three month's duration[1]. It is among the most common of all health complaints[2]. It is a major cause of activity limitation and work absence worldwide[3]. The Global Burden of Disease 2010 estimates that low back pain is amongst the top ten DALYs (disability-adjusted life years) causing diseases and injuries in the world[4]. In the developed countries like the United States, yearly prevalence of back pain varies from 10% to 56% with a lifetime prevalence of almost 80%[5]. It is the fifth most common reason for physician visits[6]. Its yearly prevalence in the developing countries is also high, varying between 36% and 64%[7-10]. Many diseases of the spine may result in back pain, and include, spinal canal stenosis, spondylolisthesis, ankylosing spondylitis, severe scoliosis, malignancy, and fracture[11]. However, most back pain is non-specific in presentation and no distinct etiology is identified in most cases[12].

The usual treatment for low back pain is non-prescription medication or non-steroidal anti-inflammatory drugs[13]. Self-care is encouraged[14]. Despite a wide range of prescription pharmacologic agents[15], non-pharmacologic medical interventions[16], and surgical procedures[17-20], most patients report only mild or moderate relief. Prognosis remains poor[21-22]. Several complementary and alternative medicine modalities are also used for its treatment, by the general population[23-24]. Yoga is a bio-psycho-social intervention that appears to be helpful in the management of this condition[25].

Yoga and Back Pain

Several large and well-designed studies support yoga's effectiveness in helping patients with chronic low back pain[26,27].

In a study involving 228 adults with chronic low back pain, three groups were studied. Patients were randomized to 12 weekly classes of yoga (n=92) or conventional stretching exercises (n=91) or self-care (n=45). At the end of 12 and 26 weeks, the yoga group were superior to those in the self-care group. Yoga was not superior to conventional stretching exercises at any time point[28]. Similar findings were reported by Saper and group[29].

Over the years, extensive trials have been published, expounding the discomfort relieving and functionality improving effects of yoga practice in patients with chronic back pain. Five smaller randomized controlled trials have validated these findings[30-34]. Similar conclusions were reached in five major randomized controlled trials[35-39]. These findings were also confirmed by several systemic reviews and meta-analysis[40-42].

The practice guidelines from the American Pain Society and the American College of Physicians[43] support yoga as an evidence-based treatment for chronic low back pain with expectation of at least moderate benefit.

Pain is the main disabling symptom, experienced by 80%-90% patients with chronic back discomfort[44]. The aim of therapeutic modalities is thus aimed primarily at reducing pain, preventing pain catastrophizing and increasing pain tolerance. Yoga has emerged as the forerunner in the treatment of pain affecting the lower back[45]. It favorably affects all parameters of pain[46]. Since pain has a strong 'mind-connection' component[47], yoga by "uncoupling" the physical sensation, from the emotional and cognitive experiences of pain, contributes to the relief process. The pain reduction persists for several months, as evidenced by post-treatment follow-ups[48-49], and pain medication usage is considerably reduced.

Yoga uses the body's own weight and earth's gravity to put the various parts of the body through a range of motion. These postures gradually increase muscle strength and joint flexibility[50-52], both in healthy individuals[53] in patients with chronic low back pain[54]. Muscular endurance is improved[55]. Yoga postures put the spine through a wide range of motions and help improve spinal alignment and bodily posture[56]. Balance is improved, and falls are reduced, especially in the elderly[57-58]. These musculoskeletal improvements also help ameliorate chronic low back pain.

Associated psychological impairments are extremely common in patients with chronic low back pain[59]. The three common comorbidities are depression, anxiety and sleep disorders[60-62]. Depression incidence is doubled in patients with chronic low back pain[63], and appears to have a bidirectional association: depression is a predictor of persistent pain and pain is a predictor of persistence of depression[64,65]. There is strong evidence from several randomized trials supporting the benefits of yoga in reducing depression[66,67]. Depression in patients with low back pain prognosticate a more refractory and longer therapeutic course and more workplace time lost[68]. The beneficial role of yoga in alleviating anxiety is also well documented[69]. Sleep disorders are also a common co-morbidity of chronic back pain[70-71], and yoga helps in improving sleep in these patients[72]. Yoga increases functionality in patients with chronic back pain[73,74]. There are documented improvements in the quality of life in these patients[75-78]. There is also a positive effect provided by a sense of belonging when attending a yoga class – resulting in an increase in emotional and tangible support[79].

Yoga practice also modulates serum brain-derived neurotrophic factor (BDNF) and serotonin levels in patients with chronic low back pain. Changes in these neuromodulators helps in the attenuation of the chronic low back pain[80].

Yoga practice not only helps ameliorate chronic low back pain but also helps rectify its associated psychological comorbidities. It is extremely cost-effective. Compliance is good[81], and the benefits are usually long lasting.

Conclusion

Yoga is well suited as an adjunctive therapy for patients with chronic low back pain.

References

1. Croft PR, Macfarlane GJ, Papageorgiou AC, et al. Outcome of low back pain in general practice: a prospective study. BMJ 1998; 316:1356–1359.
2. Rives PA, Douglass AB. Evaluation and treatment of low back pain in family practice. J Am Board Fam Pract. 2004;17: S23–31.
3. Hoy D, Christopher Bain, Gail Williams, et al. A systematic review of the global prevalence of low back pain. Arthritis & Rheumatism, 2012; 64(6) :2028–2037.

4. Murray CJL, Theo Vos, Rafael Lozano, et al. Disability-adjusted life years (DALYs) for 291 diseases and injuries in 21 regions, 1990–2010: a systematic analysis for the Global Burden of Disease Study 2010. Lancet 2012; 380: 2197–223.

5. Rubin DI. Epidemiology and risk factors for spine pain. Neurol Clin. 2007;25(2):353–371.

6. Chou R, Qaseem A, Snow V, et al. Clinical Efficacy Assessment Subcommittee of the American College of Physicians; American College of Physicians; American Pain Society Low Back Pain Guidelines Panel. Diagnosis and treatment of low back pain: a joint clinical practice guideline from the American College of Physicians and the American Pain Society. Ann Intern Med. 2007;147(7):478–91.

7. Hoy D, Toole MJ, Morgan D et al. (2003). Low back in rural Tibet. Lancet 361 225–226.

8. Cakmak A, Yucel B, Ozalcin SN, et al. (2004). The frequency and associated factors of low back pain among a younger population in Turkey. Spine 29: 1567–1572. 2004.

9. Gilgil E, Kacar C, Butun B, et al. (2005). Prevalence of low back pain in a developing urban setting. Spine 30: 1093–1098. 2005.

10. Barrero LH, Hsu YH, Terwedow H, et al. (2006). Prevalence and physical determinants of low back pain in a rural Chinese population. Spine 31 2728–2734.

11. Saper RB, Boah AR, Keosaian J, Cerrada C, Weinberg J, Sherman KJ. Comparing Once- versus Twice-Weekly Yoga Classes for Chronic Low Back Pain in Predominantly Low-Income Minorities: A Randomized Dosing Trial. Evidence-based Complementary and Alternative Medicine□: eCAM. 2013;2013:658030. doi:10.1155/2013/658030.

12. Deyo RA, Weinstein JN. Low back pain. N Engl J Med. 2001;344:363–370. doi: 10.1056/NEJM200102013440508.

13. van Tulder MW, Scholten RJPM, Koes BW, Deyo RA. Non-steroidal anti-inflammatory drugs for low-back pain. The Cochrane Database of Systematic Reviews 2000, Issue 2. Art. No.: CD000396. DOI: 10.1002/14651858.CD000396.

14. Chenot JF, Greitemann B, Kladny B, Petzke F, Pfingsten M, Schorr SG. Non-Specific Low Back Pain. Dtsch Arztebl Int. 2017 Dec 25;114(51-52):883–890. doi: 10.3238/arztebl.2017.0883.

15. (Pletcher MJ, Kertesz SG, Kohn MA, Gonzales R. Trends in opioid prescribing by race/ethnicity for patients seeking care in US emergency departments. JAMA. 2008;299:70–78.

16. Chou R, Huffman LH. Nonpharmacologic therapies for acute and chronic low back pain: a review of the evidence for an American Pain Society/American College of Physicians clinical practice guideline. Ann Intern Med. 2007;147:492–504. doi: 10.7326/0003-4819-147-7-200710020-00007.

17. Wolsko PM, Eisenberg DM, Davis RB, et al. Patterns and perceptions of care for treatment of back and neck pain: results of a national survey. Spine. 2003; 28:292-7.

18. Haldeman S, Dagenais S. A supermarket approach to the evidence-informed management of chronic low back pain. Spine J. 2008; 8:1–7.
19. Balague F, Mannion AF, Fellise F, et al. Non-specific low back pain. Lancet. 2012; 379:482–91.van Tulder et al, 2000.
20. Bogduk, 2004; Wolsko et al, 2003; Mroz TE, Norvell DC, Ecker E, Gruenberg M, Dailey A, Brodke DS. Fusion versus nonoperative management for chronic low back pain: do sociodemographic factors affect outcome? Spine (Phila Pa 1976). 2011 Oct 1;36(21 Suppl): S75-86. doi: 10.1097/BRS.0b013e31822ef68c.)
21. Carey TS, Garrett JM, Jackman AM. Beyond the good prognosis: examination of an inception cohort of patients with chronic low back pain. Spine 2000; 25:115-20,
22. Grotle M, Vollestad NK, Brox JI. Clinical course and impact of fear-avoidance beliefs in low back pain: prospective cohort study of acute and chronic low back pain II. Spine 2006; 31:1038-46.
23. Sherman KJ, Cherkin DC, Connelly MT, et al. Complementary and alternative medical therapies for chronic low back pain: What treatments are patients willing to try? BMC Complement Altern Med. 2004. July 19;4: 9.
24. Ghildayal N, Johnson PJ, Evans RL, Kreitzer MJ. Complementary and Alternative Medicine Use in the US Adult Low Back Pain Population. Global Advances in Health and Medicine. 2016;5(1):69-78. doi:10.7453/gahmj.2015.104.
25. Guzman J, Esmail R, Karjalainen K, et al. Multidisciplinary bio-psycho-social rehabilitation for chronic low back pain. Cochrane Database Syst Rev. 2002.
26. (Galantino ML, Bzdewka TM, Eissler-Russo JL, et al. The impact of modified Hatha yoga on chronic low back pain: a pilot study. Altern Ther Health Med. 2004; 10:56-9.
27. Holtzman S, Beggs RT. Yoga for chronic low back pain: A meta-analysis of randomized controlled trials. Pain Res Manag. 2013 Sep-Oct; 18(5): 267–272.
28. Sherman KJ, Cherkin DC, Wellman RD, et al. A Randomized Trial Comparing Yoga, Stretching, and a Self-care Book for Chronic Low Back Pain. Archives of Internal Medicine. 2011;171(22):2019-2026. doi:10.1001/archinternmed.2011.524.
29. Saper RB, Boah AR, Keosaian J, Cerrada C, Weinberg J, Sherman KJ. Comparing Once- versus Twice-Weekly Yoga Classes for Chronic Low Back Pain in Predominantly Low Income Minorities: A Randomized Dosing Trial. Evidence-based Complementary and Alternative Medicine: eCAM. 2013;2013:658030. doi:10.1155/2013/658030.
30. Williams KA, Petronis J, Smith D, Goodrich D, Wu J, Ravi N, Doyle EJ Jr, Gregory JR, Munoz KM, Gross R, Steinberg L. Effect of Iyengar yoga therapy for chronic low back pain. Pain. 2005;115:107–117. doi: 10.1016/j.pain.2005.02.016.
31. Saper RB, Sherman KJ, Cullum-Dugan D, Davis RB, Phillips RS, Culpepper L. Yoga for chronic low back pain in a predominantly minority

population: a pilot randomized controlled trial. Altern Ther Health Med. 2009;15(6):18–27.

32. Galantino ML, Bzdewka TM, Eissler-Russo JL, Holbrook ML, Mogck EP, Geigle P, Farrar JT. The impact of modified Hatha yoga on chronic low back pain: a pilot study. Altern Ther Health Med. 2004;10:56–59.

33. Cox H, Tilbrook H, Aplin J, Semlyen A, Torgerson D, Trewhela A, Watt I. A randomised controlled trial of yoga for the treatment of chronic low back pain: results of a pilot study. Complement Ther Clin Pract. 2010;16:187–193. doi: 10.1016/j.ctcp.2010.05.007.

34. Tekur P, Nagarathna R, Chametcha S, Hankey A, Nagendra HR. A comprehensive yoga programs improves pain, anxiety and depression in chronic low back pain patients more than exercise: an RCT. Complement Ther Med. 2012;20:107–118. doi: 10.1016/j.ctim.2011.12.009.) support yoga's effectiveness for reducing pain and improving function in adults with cLBP.

35. Sherman KJ, Cherkin DC, Erro J, Miglioretti DL, Deyo RA. Comparing yoga, exercise, and a self-care book for chronic low back pain: a randomized, controlled trial. Ann Intern Med. 2005;143:849–856. doi: 10.7326/0003-4819-143-12-200512200-00003.

36. Williams K, Abildso C, Steinberg L, Doyle E, Epstein B, Smith D, Hobbs G, Gross R, Kelley G, Cooper L. Evaluation of the effectiveness and efficacy of Iyengar yoga therapy on chronic low back pain. Spine. 2009;34:2066–2076. doi: 10.1097/BRS.0b013e3181b315cc.

37. Sherman KJ, Cherkin DC, Wellman RD, Cook AJ, Hawkes RJ, Delaney K, Deyo RA. A randomized trial comparing yoga, stretching, and a self-care book for chronic low back pain. Arch Intern Med. 2011;171(22):2019–2026. doi: 10.1001/archinternmed.2011.524.

38. Tilbrook HE, Cox H, Hewitt CE, Kang'ombe AR, Chuang LH, Jayakody S, Aplin JD, Semlyen A, Trewhela A, Watt I, Torgerson DJ. Yoga for chronic low back pain: a randomized trial. Ann Intern Med. 2011;155(9):569–578. doi: 10.7326/0003-4819-155-9-201111010-00003.

39. Saper RB, Boah AR, Keosaian J, Cerrada C, Weinberg J, Sherman KJ. Comparing once- versus twice-weekly yoga classes for chronic low back pain in predominantly low income minorities: a randomized dosing trial. Evid Based Complement Alternat Med. 2013;2013:658030.

40. Posadzki P, Ernst E. Yoga for low back pain: a systematic review of randomized clinical trials. Clin Rheumatol. 2011;30(9):1257–1262. doi: 10.1007/s10067-011-1764-8.

41. Bussing A, Ostermann T, Ludtke R, Michalsen A. Effects of yoga interventions on pain and pain-associated disability: a meta-analysis. J Pain. 2012;13:1–9.

42. Cramer H, Lauche R, Haller H, Dobos G. A systematic review and meta-analysis of yoga for low back pain. Clin J Pain. 2013;29(5):450–460. doi: 10.1097/AJP.0b013e31825e1492.

43. Chou R, Huffman LH. Nonpharmacologic therapies for acute and chronic low back pain: a review of the evidence for an American Pain Society/American College of Physicians clinical practice guideline. Ann

Intern Med. 2007;147:492–504. doi: 10.7326/0003-4819-147-7-200710020-00007.

44. Kovacs FM, Abraira V, Zamora J, et al. Spanish Back Pain Research Network. The transition from acute to subacute and chronic low back pain: A study based on determinants of quality of life and prediction of chronic disability. Spine (Phila Pa 1976) 2005; 30:1786–92.

45. Evans DD, Carter M, Panico R, et al. Characteristics and predictors of short-term outcomes in individuals self-selecting yoga or physical therapy for treatment of chronic low back pain. PM R. 2010; 2:1006–1015.

46. Tilbrook HE, Cox H, Hewitt CE, et al. Yoga for chronic low back pain. Ann Intern Med. 2011; 155:569–78.

47. Kabat-Zinn J, Lipworth L, Burney R, et al. Four-Year Follow-up of a meditation-based program for the self-regulation of chronic pain: Treatment outcomes and compliance. Clin J Pain. 1986; 2:159–73.

48. Jacobs BP, Mehling W, Avins AL, et al. Feasibility of conducting a clinical trial on Hatha yoga for chronic low back pain: methodological lessons. Altern Ther Health Med. 2004; 10:80-3.

49. Sherman KJ, Daniel C. Cherkin, Janet Erro, et al. Comparing Yoga, Exercise, and a Self-Care Book for Chronic Low Back Pain: A Randomized, Controlled Trial. Ann Intern Med. 2005;143(12):849-856.

50. Roland KP, Jakobi JM, Jones GR. Does yoga engender fitness in older adults? A critical review. J Aging Phys Act. 2011; 19:62–79. ; 23.

51. Field T. Yoga clinical research review. Complement Ther Clin Pract. 2011; 17:1–8.

52. Caren Lau, Ruby Yu, Jean Woo. Effects of a 12-Week Hatha Yoga Intervention on Cardiorespiratory Endurance, Muscular Strength and Endurance, and Flexibility in Hong Kong Chinese Adults: A Controlled Clinical Trial. Evid Based Complement Alternat Med. 2015; 2015: 958727.

53. Tran M. D., Holly R. G., Lashbrook J., Amsterdam E. A. Effects of hatha yoga practice on the health-related aspects of physical fitness. Preventive Cardiology. 2001;4(4):165–170.

54. Tekur P, Chametcha S, Hongasandra RN, et al. Effect of yoga on quality of life of CLBP patients: A randomized control study. Int J Yoga. 2010;3:10–17.

55. Chen K. M., Chen M. H., Hong S. M., et al. Physical fitness of older adults in senior activity centres after 24-week silver yoga exercises. Journal of Clinical Nursing. 2008;17(19):2634–2646.

56. Gail A. Greendale, Mei-Hua Huang, Arun S. Karlamangla, et al. Yoga decreases kyphosis in senior women and men with adult onset hyperkyphosis: results of a randomized controlled trial. J Am Geriatr Soc. 2009 Sep; 57(9): 1569–1579.

57. Vaughan P Nicholson, Mark R McKean, and Brendan J Burkett. Twelve weeks of BodyBalance® training improved balance and functional task performance in middle-aged and older adults. Clin Interv Aging. 2014; 9: 1895–1904.

58. Saravanakumar P, Higgins IJ, van der Riet PJ, et al. The influence of tai chi and yoga on balance and falls in a residential care setting: A randomised controlled trial. Contemp Nurse. 2014;48(1):76-87.

59. Demyttenaere K, Bruffaerts R, Lee S, et al. Mental disorders among persons with chronic back or neck pain: results from the World Mental Health Surveys. Pain. 2007 Jun;129(3):332-42.; Linton SJ. A review of psychological risk factors in back and neck pain. Spine. 2000; 25:1148–56.

60. Long-term medical conditions and major depression in a Canadian population study at waves 1 and 2. J Affect Disord. 2001; 63:35–41.

61. Newcomer KL, Shelerud RA, Vickers Douglas KS, et al. Anxiety levels, fear-avoidance beliefs, and disability levels at baseline and at 1 year among subjects with acute and chronic low back pain. PM R 2010; 2:514–20.

62. Bahouq H, Allali F, Rkain H, et al. Prevalence and severity of insomnia in chronic low back pain patients. Rheumatol Int. 2013; 33:1277–81.

63. Patten SB. Long-term medical conditions and major depression in a Canadian population study at waves 1 and 2. J Affect Disord. 2001; 63:35–41.

64. Ohayon MM, Schatzberg AF (2003) Using chronic pain to predict depressive morbidity in the general population. Arch Gen Psychiatry 60: 39–47.

65. Saito T, Kai I, Takizawa A. Effects of a program to prevent social isolation on loneliness, depression, and subjective well-being of older adults: a randomized trial among older migrants in Japan. Arch Gerontol Geriatr 2012; 55: 539–54.

66. Kinser PA, Lisa Goehler, Ann Gill Taylor. How Might Yoga Help Depression? A Neurobiological Perspective. Explore (NY). 2012 Mar 1; 8(2): 118–126.

67. Prathikanti S, Rivera R, Cochran A, Tungol JG, Fayazmanesh N, Weinmann E. Treating major depression with yoga: A prospective, randomized, controlled pilot trial. Subramanian SK, ed. PLoS ONE. 2017;12(3):e0173869.

68. Bair MJ, Robinson RL, Katon W, et al. Depression and pain comorbidity: a literature review. Arch Intern Med. 2003 Nov 10;163(20):2433-45.

69. Hofmann SG, Curtiss J, Khalsa SB, et al. Yoga for generalized anxiety disorder: design of a randomized controlled clinical trial. Contemp Clin Trials. 2015 Aug 6; 44:70-76.

70. Bahouq H, Allali F, Rkain H, et al. Prevalence and severity of insomnia in chronic low back pain patients. Rheumatol Int. 2013; 33:1277–81.

71. Kathi L. Heffner, Christopher R. France, Zina Trost, et al. Chronic Low Back Pain, Sleep Disturbance, and Interleukin-6. Clin J Pain. 2011 Jan; 27(1): 35–41.

72. Balasubramaniam M, Shirley Telles, P. Murali Doraiswamy. Yoga on Our Minds: A Systematic Review of Yoga for Neuropsychiatric Disorders. Front Psychiatry. 2012; 3: 117.

73. Telles S, Kalkuni V Naveen, Vaishali Gaur, et al. Effect of one week of yoga on function and severity in rheumatoid arthritis. BMC Res Notes. 2011; 4: 118.

74. Holtzman S, Beggs RT. Yoga for chronic low back pain: A meta-analysis of randomized controlled trials. Pain Res Manag. 2013 Sep-Oct; 18(5): 267–272.

75. Oken BS, Zajdel D, Kishiyama S, et al. Randomized, controlled, six-month trial of yoga in healthy seniors: effects on cognition and quality of life. Altern Ther Health Med. 2006;12(1):40–47.

76. Williams K, Abildso C, Steinberg L, Doyle E, Epstein B, et al. Evaluation of the effectiveness and efficacy of Iyengar yoga therapy on chronic low back pain. Spine (Phila Pa 1976) 2009;34:2066–2076.

77. Tekur P, Chametcha S, Hongasandra RN, et al. Effect of yoga on quality of life of CLBP patients: A randomized control study. Int J Yoga. 2010;3:10–17.

78. Banth S, Maryam Didehdar Ardebil. Effectiveness of mindfulness meditation on pain and quality of life of patients with chronic low back pain. Int J Yoga. 2015 Jul-Dec;8(2):128-33.

79. Wren AA, Wright MA, Carson JW, et al. Yoga for persistent pain: New findings and directions for an ancient practice. Pain. 2011; 152:477–80.

80. Lee M, Moon W, Kim J. Effect of yoga on pain, brain-derived neurotrophic factor, and serotonin in premenopausal women with chronic low back pain. Evid Based Complement Alternat Med. 2014;2014:203173.

81. Caren Lau, Ruby Yu, Jean Woo. Effects of a 12-Week Hatha Yoga Intervention on Cardiorespiratory Endurance, Muscular Strength and Endurance, and Flexibility in Hong Kong Chinese Adults: A Controlled Clinical Trial. Evid Based Complement Alternat Med. 2015; 2015: 958727.

Cancer

Cancer is a major public health problem worldwide[1-5]. According to the American Cancer Society, it is estimated that in 2017, there will be 688,780 new cancer cases diagnosed and 600,920 cancer deaths in the US[6]. It continues to be the second leading cause of death in the USA[6]. The statistics are also dismal for the entire world - in 2012, there were 14.1 million new cases of cancer diagnosed, and 32.6 million people were living with cancer[7]. In 2015, available data indicates that cancer caused 8.8 million deaths and was the second leading cause of death, globally[8]. It is estimated that in 2030, new cancer cases will increase to almost 21.7 million and cancer deaths to 13 million, around the world[9]. The period encompassing the diagnosis of cancer, its treatment, and the post treatment rehabilitation, is often associated with a significant disruption in a patient's life. This entire period may be complicated by a litany of distressing factors, and these include anxiety, stress, and depression[10]. Fatigue and insomnia also contribute greatly to the overall discomfort[11,12]. Pain, both acute and chronic, is also common during this stage[13-16]. Chemotherapy may further bring disturbing nausea and vomiting[17]. These symptoms, unfortunately, often occur concomitantly, and result in a significant reduction in the quality of life of these patients [18-20]. A host of non-pharmacological therapeutic interventions have been tried to alleviate the cancer discomfort and its treatment related 'dis-eases', with limited success[21-25]. Yoga therapy has been demonstrating an increasing potential benefit in improving these cancer-related physical and emotional issues, and greatly improving the quality of life of these patients[26,27].

Yoga and Cancer

Symptoms of anxiety are part of everyone's life and are common in the general population,[28] but pathological anxiety is significantly more common[29,30] and often under-diagnosed in cancer patients[31]. Significant anxiety may affect from 2% to 14% of patients with advanced cancer[32-34]. Its presence is associated with a subjective increase in other symptoms and these patients experience decreased physical functioning [35]. Anxiety also results in a poorer quality of life in these patients[36]. Survival time is decreased[37]. Yoga has beneficial effects in the complementary treatment of anxiety[38]. Meditation helps decrease anxiety in the cancer patients[39,40]. Yoga exercise also helps ameliorate cancer related anxiety[41-43].

Depression is also common in cancer patients[44], with prevalence rates of 13% to 40%[45,46]. These rates are much higher than that seen in the general population[47]. About 20% to 30% of breast cancer patients experience severe depression[48]. Depressed cancer patients have a decreased quality of life[49.] The negative effect on mortality has also been documented[50,51]. Unfortunately, despite the availability of excellent therapeutic pharmaceuticals for this ailment, antidepressant therapy is often associated with non-efficacy, drug resistance[52] polypharmacy[53] non-compliance, frequent relapses and a high cost[54-56].

Several studies have provided persuasive evidence attesting to the benefits of yoga therapy in patients with depression[57-60]. Attenuation of depression has also been noted in patients with cancer, specially breast cancer, in several clinical trials[61-63]. A recent Cochrane meta-analysis of 23 studies involving 2166 participants, concluded that a moderate quality evidence exists in supporting the use of yoga for a therapeutic reduction in depression, anxiety and fatigue, when compared with other psychosocial/educational interventions, in patients with breast cancer[64]. Reduction of depression has also been noted in other cancers[65]. Interestingly, emotional benefits with yoga practice have also been seen in cancer caregivers with yoga therapy[66].

Pain in cancer is common[67], and often the most feared symptom[68]. Pain may be due to the cancer itself, or its treatments, which may include surgery, chemotherapy and radiotherapy[69]. It is estimated that up to 20% of cancer patients are unable to find pain relief with conventional treatment[70]. When the malignant disease is advanced, almost 70% of patients may be unable to get rid of the pain[71]. Complimentary therapies are often resorted to by these patients[72,73]. Some studies have demonstrated benefits of yoga in pain reduction in these patients[74,75].

Nausea and vomiting is also a common side effect of cancer chemotherapy[76], and can be very distressing[77-81]. It remains one of the most difficult of all side effects to treat in these patients[82,83]. It greatly reduces the quality of life[84]. Its appearance may also lead to a dangerous refusal to continue essential cancer treatment[85].

Yoga therapy has also been studied in these patients, as a complementary modality. A small study in 2007, reported a significant decrease in post-chemotherapy-induced nausea frequency, nausea severity, and intensity of anticipatory nausea and vomiting in patients practicing yoga when compared with the non-yoga control group[86]. However, a recent 8-week study did not demonstrate a benefit stemming from the practice of yoga in ameliorating symptoms of nausea and vomiting related to cancer chemotherapy[87].

Patients with cancer frequently experience significant fatigue[88,89]. The prevalence rates may be as high as 75% in these patients[90]. Besides the cancer[91], treatment with chemotherapy and radiotherapy is often associated with fatigue and this further reduces the patient's quality of life[92-94]. In one study, a quarter of all cancer patients experienced severe fatigue during a six month follow up, during palliative treatment[95]. Fatigue in cancer patients is also quite persistent, and up to one third of them may experience it for up to 10 years after the cancer diagnosis[96]. Cancer-related fatigue is the most important cause of a decreased quality of life in these patients[97]. It's presence also appears to prognosticate a reduced survival[98].

Physical exercise has been suggested to combat this often stubborn and persistent symptom[99]. Yoga has also been successfully tried. Besides incorporating exercise, yoga diminishes many adverse psychological emotions in cancer patients, further attenuating the feelings of fatigue[100]. Many yoga participants also experience improved sleep patterns[101]. A Cochrane review, after performing a meta-analysis of 23 studies involving 2166 participants, concluded that yoga practice presented a moderate-quality evidence in reducing fatigue and sleep disturbances when compared with no therapy, in cancer patients[102].

Poor quality of sleep is extremely common in cancer patients[103,104], but often ignored[105]. The causes are multifactorial and include cancer related symptoms, treatment side effects, and a host of associated emotional factors[106-108]. The positive benefits of yoga in establishing better sleep in cancer patients has been reported in some studies[109,110]. A recent trial involving 410 patients demonstrated that the group participating in yoga, noticed an improvement in several sleep parameters, including reduction in postintervention medication use, when compared with standard care participants[111]. Yoga appears to play a beneficial role in the management of sleep disturbances in cancer patients.

The World Health Organization defines health as a state of complete physical, mental, and social well-being and not merely the absence of disease or infirmity[112]. Quality of life (QOL) or health – is an individual's perceived physical and mental health, and can be measured by several means, including self-reported questionnaires[113-115], such as the Health-related quality of life (HRQOL)[116], SF-36[117], EuroQol[118], and WHOQOL[119]. Quality of life is becoming an important consideration and its improvement, one of the therapeutic goals, in the treatment of many diseases, including cancer[120]. Quality of life in cancer, is the physical, emotional, social and functional well-being and perceived symptom burden, from a patient's point of view[121]. Cancer diagnosis, treatment and survival greatly affect the QOL in these patients [122]. Several demographic risk factors also are related to cancer-related QOL[123]. QOL also appears to prognosticate survival in many cancers[124-126].

Yoga can improve the quality of life in cancer patients[127]. Several studies have shown that women with breast cancer realize a marked improvement in quality of life scores and emotional well-being with yoga therapy[128-131]. The beneficial effect of yoga on the quality of life has also been noted in other cancers[132-134].

Conclusion

Yoga therapy, has a viable, evidence based role, as a complementary therapeutic modality, for alleviating several extremely distressing symptoms experienced by cancer patients.

References

1. Ries LAG, Smith MA, Gurney JG. eds, et al. 2013. Cancer Incidence and Survival among Children and Adolescents: United States SEER Program 1975-1995. NIH Pub. No. 99-4649. Bethesda, MD: National Institutes of Health; 1999.
2. Herbst RS, Heymach JV, Lippman SM. 2008. Lung cancer. N. Engl. J. Med. 359, 1367–1380.
3. Kuipers EJ, Grady WM, Lieberman D, et al. COLORECTAL CANCER. Nature reviews Disease primers. 2015;1:15065. doi:10.1038/nrdp.2015.65.
4. Radoi L., Luce D. A review of risk factors for oral cavity cancer: the importance of a standardized case definition. Commun. Dent. Oral. Epidemiol. 2013;109:e78–e91.

5. Ryerson AB, Eheman CR, Altekruse SF, et al. Annual Report to the Nation on the Status of Cancer, 1975–2012, Featuring the Increasing Incidence of Liver Cancer. Cancer. 2016;122(9):1312-1337. doi:10.1002/cncr.29936.

6. https://www.cancer.org/research/cancer-facts-statistics/all-cancer-facts-figures/cancer-facts-figures-2017.html (accessed May 24, 2017).

7. Ferlay J, Soerjomataram I, Ervik M, et al. globocan 2012: Estimated Cancer Incidence and Mortality Worldwide in 2012 [Web resource] Lyon, France: International Agency for Research on Cancer; 2012. Ver 1.0.

8. www.who.in/mediacenter/factsheets/fs297/en(accessed May 24, 2017).

9. https: // www.cancer.org/research/cancer-facts-statistics/global.html(accessed May 12, 2017)

10. Caraceni A, Portenoy RK. A working group of the IASP Task Force on Cancer Pain. An international survey of cancer pain characteristics and syndromes. Pain. 1999;82:263–74

11. Goedendorp MM, Gielissen MF, Verhagen CA, et al. Development of fatigue in cancer survivors: a prospective follow-up study from diagnosis into the year after treatment. J Pain Symptom Manag. 2013;45:213–222.

12. Ancoli-Israel S. Recognition and treatment of sleep disturbances in cancer. J Clin Oncol. 2009;27:5864–6.

13. Daut RL, Cleeland CS. The prevalence and severity of pain in cancer. Cancer. 1982;50:1913–8.

14. Strang P. Cancer pain - A provoker of emotional, social and existential distress. Acta Oncol. 1983;37:641–4.

15. Grossman SA. Undertreatment of cancer pain: Barriers and remedies. Support Care Cancer. 1993;1:74–8.

16. Ripamonti C, Dickerson ED. Strategies for the treatment of cancer pain in the new millennium. Drugs. 2001;61:955–77.

17. Iihara H, Fujii H, Yoshimi C, et al. Control of chemotherapy-induced nausea in patients receiving outpatient cancer chemotherapy. International Journal of Clinical Oncology. 2016;21:409-418.

18. Allard P, Maunsell E, Labbe J, Dorval M. Educational interventions to improve cancer pain control: A systematic review. J Palliat Med. 2001;4:191–203.

19. Conroy T, Marchal F, Blazeby JM. Quality of life in patients with oesophageal and gastric cancer: an overview. Oncology. 2006;70:391–402.

20. Costanzo ES, Lutgendorf SK, Mattes ML, et al. Adjusting to life after treatment: distress and quality of life following treatment for breast cancer. British Journal of Cancer. 2007;97(12):1625–1631.

21. Menefee LA, Monti DA. Nonpharmacologic and complementary approaches to cancer pain management. J Am Osteopath Assoc. 2005;105:S15–20.

22. Goldstein MS, Brown ER, Ballard-Barbash R, Morgenstern H, Bastani R, Lee J, et al. The use of complementary and alternative medicine among Californian adults with and without cancer. Evid Based Complement Altern Med. 2005;2:557–65.

23. Smith KB, Pukall CF. An evidence-based review of yoga as a complementary intervention for patients with cancer. Psychooncology. 2009 May;18(5):465-75. doi: 10.1002/pon.1411.

24. Anderson JG, Taylor AG. Use of complementary therapies for cancer symptom management: Results of the 2007 national health interview survey. Journal of Alternative and Complementary Medicine. 2012;18(3):235–41.

25. Chandwani KD, Ryan JL, Peppone LJ, Janelsins MM, Sprod LK, Devine K, et al. Cancer-related stress and complementary and alternative medicine: A review. Evidence-based Complementary and Alternative Medicine. 2012;979213.

26. Vadiraja SH, Rao MR, Nagendra RH, et al. Effects of yoga on symptom management in breast cancer patients: A randomized controlled trial. Int J Yoga. 2009 Jul;2(2):73-9.

27. Greenlee H, DuPont-Reyes MJ, Balneaves LG, et al. Clinical practice guidelines on the evidence-based use of integrative therapies during and after breast cancer treatment. CA Cancer J Clin. 2017 May 6;67(3):194-232.

28. Karsnitz D, Ward S. Spectrum of anxiety disorders: diagnosis and pharmacologic treatment. J Midwifery Womens Health. 2011;56:266–281.

29. Teunissen SCCM, de Graeff A, Voest EE, de Hass JCJM. Are anxiety and depressed mood related to physical symptom burden? A study in hospitalized advanced cancer patients. Palliat Med. 2007;21:341–346.

30. Kolva E, Rosenfeld B, Pessin H, Breitbart W, Brescia R. Anxiety in Terminally Ill Cancer Patients. Journal of pain and symptom management. 2011;42(5):691-701.

31. Mitchell AJ, Ferguson DW, Gill J, et al. Depression and anxiety in long-term cancer survivors compared with spouses and healthy controls: A systematic review and meta-analysis. Lancet Oncol. 2013;14:721–732.

32. Kissane DW, Grabsch B, Love A, et al. Psychiatric disorder in women with early stage and advanced breast cancer: a comparative analysis. Aust N Z J Psychiatry. 2004;38:320–326.

33. Kadan-Lottick NS, Vanderwerker LC, Block SD, Zhang B, Prigerson HG. Psychiatric disorders and mental health service use in patients with advanced cancer. Cancer. 2005;104:2872–2881.

34. Miovic M, Block S. Psychiatric disorders in advanced cancer. Cancer. 2007;15(110):1665–1676.

35. Aass N, Fossa SD, Dahl AA, et al. Prevalence of anxiety and depression in cancer patients seen at the Norwegian Radium Hospital. Eur J Cancer. 1997;33:1597–1604.

36. Brown LF, Kroenke K, Theobald DE, et al. The association of depression and anxiety with health-related quality of life in cancer patients with depression and/or pain. Psychooncology. 2010;19:734–741.

37. Groenvold M, Petersen MA, Idler E, et al. Psychological distress and fatigue predicted recurrence and survival in primary breast cancer patients. Breast Cancer Res Treat. 2007;105:209–219.

38. Streeter CC, Whitfield TH, Owen L, et al. Effects of Yoga Versus Walking on Mood, Anxiety, and Brain GABA Levels: A Randomized Controlled MRS Study. Journal of Alternative and Complementary Medicine. 2010;16(11):1145-1152.

39. Kim YH, Kim HJ, Ahn SD, Seo YJ, Kim SH. Effects of meditation on anxiety, depression, fatigue, and quality of life of women undergoing

radiation therapy for breast cancer. Complement Ther Med. 2013;21:379-387.

40. Carlson LE, Doll R, Stephen J, et al. Randomized controlled trial of mindfulness-based cancer recovery versus supportive expressive group therapy for distressed survivors of breast cancer. J Clin Oncol. 2013;31:3119-3126.

41. Taso CJ, Lin HS, Lin WL, Chen SM, Huang WT, Chen SW. The effect of yoga exercise on improving depression, anxiety, and fatigue in women with breast cancer: a randomized controlled trial. J Nurs Res. 2014;22:155-164.

42. Dhruva A, Miaskowski C, Abrams D, et al. Yoga breathing for cancer chemotherapy-associated symptoms and quality of life: results of a pilot randomized controlled trial. J Alternat Complement Med. 2012;18:473-479.

43. Pruthi S, Stan DL, Jenkins SM, et al. A randomized controlled pilot study assessing feasibility and impact of yoga practice on quality of life, mood, and perceived stress in women with newly diagnosed breast cancer. Glob Adv Health Med. 2012;1:30-35.

44. Raison CL, Miller AH. Depression in cancer: new developments regarding diagnosis and treatment. Biol Psychiatry. 2003;54:283–294.

45. Coyne JC, Stefanek M, Palmer SC. Psychotherapy and survival in cancer: the conflict between hope and evidence. Psychol Bull 2007;133:367–94.

46. Bottino SMB, Fraguas R, Gattaz WF. Depressão e cancer [[Depression and cancer]. Rev Psiq Clin. 2009; 36:109–15.

47. Massie MJ. Prevalence of depression is patients with cancer. J Natl Cancer Inst Monogr. 2004:57–71.

48. Fann JR, Thomas-Rich AM, Katon WJ, Cowley D, Pepping M, McGregor BA, Gralow J. Major depression after breast cancer: a review of epidemiology and treatment. Gen Hosp Psychiatry. 2008;30:112–126.

49. Grabsch B, Clarke DM, Love A, et al. Psychological morbidity and quality of life in women with advanced breast cancer: A cross-sectional survey. Palliat Support Care. 2006;4:47–56.

50. Onitilo AA, Nietert PJ, Egede LE. Effect of depression on all-cause mortality in adults with cancer and differential effects by cancer site. Gen Hosp Psych. 2006;28:396–402.

51. Pirl WF, Greer JA, Traeger L, et al. Depression and Survival in Metastatic Non–Small-Cell Lung Cancer: Effects of Early Palliative Care. Journal of Clinical Oncology. 2012;30(12):1310-1315.

52. Al-Harbi KS. Treatment-resistant depression: therapeutic trends, challenges, and future directions. Patient Prefer Adherence. 2012;6:369–388.

53. Covadonga M. Díaz-Caneja Ana Espliego Mara Parellada Celso Arango Carmen Moreno. Polypharmacy with antidepressants in children and adolescents. Int J Neuropsychopharmacol (2014) 17 (7).

54. Keller MB. McCullough JP. Klein DN, et al. A comparison of nefazodone, the cognitive behavioral–analysis system of psychotherapy, and their combination for the treatment of chronic depression. N Engl J Med. 2000;342(20):1462–1470.

55. Van H. L., Dekker J., Peen J., Van Aalst G., Schoevers R. A. Identifying patients at risk of complete nonresponse in the outpatient treatment of depression. Psychotherapy and Psychosomatics. 2008;77(6):358–364.

56. Santarsieri D, Schwartz TL. Antidepressant efficacy and side-effect burden: a quick guide for clinicians. Drugs Context. 2015 Oct 8;4: 212290.

57. Saeed SA, Antonacci DJ, Bloch RM. Exercise, yoga, and meditation for depressive and anxiety disorders. Am Fam Physician. 2010 Apr 15;81(8):981-6.

58. Uebelacker LA, Broughton MK. Yoga for Depression and Anxiety: A Review of Published Research and Implications for Healthcare Providers. R I Med J (2013). 2016 Mar 1;99(3):20-2.

59. Prathikanti S, Rivera R, Cochran A, Tungol JG, Fayazmanesh N, Weinmann E. Treating major depression with yoga: A prospective, randomized, controlled pilot trial. Subramanian SK, ed. PLoS ONE. 2017;12(3): e0173869.

60. Streeter CC, Gerberg PL, Whitfield TH, et al. Treatment of Major Depressive Disorder with Iyengar Yoga and Coherent Breathing: A Randomized Controlled Dosing Study. Journal of Alternative and Complementary Medicine. 2017;23(3):201-207.

61. Rao RM, Nagendra HR, Raghuram N, Vinay C, Chandrashekara S, Gopinath KS, Srinath BS. Influence of yoga on mood states, distress, quality of life and immune outcomes in early stage breast cancer patients undergoing surgery. Int J Yoga. 2008 Jan;1(1):11-20.

62. Rao RM, Raghuram N, Nagendra HR, et al. Effects of an integrated yoga program on self-reported depression scores in breast cancer patients undergoing conventional treatment: a randomized controlled trial. Indian J Palliat Care. 2015;21:174-181.

63. Taylor TR, Barrow J, Makambi K, et al. A Restorative Yoga Intervention for African-American Breast Cancer Survivors: a Pilot Study. J Racial Ethn Health Disparities. 2017 Apr 14.

64. Cramer H, Lauche R, Klose P, et al. Yoga for improving health-related quality of life, mental health and cancer-related symptoms in women diagnosed with breast cancer. Cochrane Database Syst Rev. 2017 Jan 3;1:CD010802.

65. Danhauer SC, Tooze JA, Farmer DF, Campbell CR, McQuellon RP, Barrett R, Miller BE. Restorative yoga for women with ovarian or breast cancer: findings from a pilot study. J Soc Integr Oncol. 2008;6(2):47–58.

66. Milbury K, Mallaiah S, Lopez G, et al. Vivekananda Yoga Program for Patients with Advanced Lung Cancer and Their Family Caregivers. Integr Cancer Ther. 2015 Sep;14(5):446-51.

67. van den Beuken-van Everdingen MH, de Rijke JM, Kessels AG, Schouten HC, van Kleef M. Patijn J. Prevalence of pain in patients with cancer: a systematic review of the past 40 years. Ann. Oncol. 2007;18:1437–1449.

68. Breitbart W. S., Park J., Katz A. M. Psycho-Oncology. 2nd. New York, NY, USA: Oxford University Press; 2010.

69. cancer.org/treatment/treatments-and-side-effects/physical-side-effects/pain/facts-about-cancer-pain.html (accessed May 24, 2017).

70. Gupta N., Patel F. D., Kapoor R., Sharma S. C. Pain management in cancer. Internet Journal of Pain, Symptom Control and Palliative Care. 2007;5(1):83–89.

71. Deandrea S, Montanari M, Moja L. Apolone G. Prevalence of undertreatment in cancer pain. A review of published literature. Ann. Oncol. 2008;19:1985–1991.

72. Wanchai A, Armer JM, Stewart BR. Complementary and alternative medicine use among women with breast cancer: a systematic review. Clin J Oncol Nurs. 2010;14:E45–55.

73. Thomas EM, Weiss SM. Nonpharmacological interventions with chronic cancer pain in adults. Cancer Control. 2000;7:157–64.

74. Carson JW, Carson KM, Porter LS, Keefe FJ, Shaw H, Miller JM. Yoga for women with metastatic breast cancer: results from a pilot study. J Pain Symptom Manage. 2007;33:331–41.

75. Galantino ML, Greene L, Archetto B, Baumgartner M, Hassall P, Murphy JK, et al. A qualitative exploration of the impact of yoga on breast cancer survivors with aromatase inhibitor-associated arthralgias. Explore (NY) 2012;8:40–7.

76. Andrews PL, Axelsson M, Franklin C, Holmgren S. The emetic reflex in a reptile (Crocodylus porosus) J. Exp. Biol. 2000;203:1625–1632.

77. Miller F. Nausea and vomiting in pregnancy: the problem of perception-- is it really a disease? American Journal of Obstetrics and Gynecology. 2002;186(5 Suppl):S182–S183.

78. Borison HL, MacCarthy LE. Neuropharmacologic mechanisms of emesis. In: Laszlo J, editor. Antiemetics and Cancer Chemotherapy. Baltimore: Williams and Wilkins; 1983. pp. 6–20.

79. Passik SD, Kirsh KL, Rosenfeld B, McDonald MV, Theobald DE. The changeable nature of patients' fear regarding chemotherapy: implications for palliative care. J Pain Symptom Manag. 2001;21:113–120.

80. Sun CC, Bodurka DC, Weaver CB, Rasu R, Wolf JK, Bevers MW, Smith JA, Wharton JT, Rubenstein EB. Rankings and symptom assessments of side effects from chemotherapy: insights from experienced patients with ovarian cancer. Support Care Cancer. 2005;13:219–227.

81. Wagland R, Richardson A, Armes J, Hankins M, Lennan E, Griffiths P (2014) Treatment-related problems experienced by cancer patients undergoing chemotherapy: a scoping review. Eur J Cancer Care. 2015 Sep;24(5):605-17.

82. Herrstedt, J. and Dombernowsky, P. (2007), Anti-Emetic Therapy in Cancer Chemotherapy: Current Status. Basic & Clinical Pharmacology & Toxicology, 101: 143–150.

83. Escobar Y, Cajaraville G, Virizuela JA, et al. Incidence of chemotherapy-induced nausea and vomiting with moderately emetogenic chemotherapy: ADVICE (Actual Data of Vomiting Incidence by Chemotherapy Evaluation) study. Supportive Care in Cancer. 2015;23(9):2833-2840.

84. Ballatori E, Roila F, Ruggeri B, Betti M, Sarti S, Soru G, Cruciani G, Di Maio M, Andrea B, Deuson RR. The impact of chemotherapy-induced nausea and vomiting on health-related quality of life. Support Care Cancer. 2007;15:179–185.

85. Vidall C, Dielenseger P, Farrell C, Lennan E, Muxagata P, Fernandez-Ortega P, Paradies K. Evidence-based management of chemotherapy-induced nausea and vomiting: a position statement from a European cancer nursing forum. Ecancermedicalsci. 2011;5:211.

86. Raghavendra RM, Nagarathna R, Nagendra HR,et al. Raghavendra RM, Nagarathna R, Nagendra HR, et al. Effects of an integrated yoga programme on chemotherapy-induced nausea and emesis in breast cancer patients. Eur J Cancer Care (Engl) 2007;16(6):462–474.
87. Anestin AS, Dupuis G, Lanctôt D, Bali M. The Effects of the Bali Yoga Program for Breast Cancer Patients on Chemotherapy-Induced Nausea and Vomiting: Results of a Partially Randomized and Blinded Controlled Trial. J Evid Based Complementary Altern Med. 2017 Jan 1:2156587217706617.
88. De Raaf PJ, De Klerk C, Timman R, et al. Differences in fatigue experiences among patients with advanced cancer, cancer survivors, and the general population. J Pain Symptom Manag. 2012;44:823–830.
89. Goedendorp MM, Gielissen MF, Verhagen CA, et al. Development of fatigue in cancer survivors: a prospective follow-up study from diagnosis into the year after treatment. J Pain Symptom Manag. 2013;45:213–222.
90. Curt GA, Breitbart W, Cella D, et al. Impact of cancer-related fatigue on the lives of patients: new findings from the Fatigue Coalition. Oncologist. 2000;5(5):353–60.
91. Spichiger E, Muller-Frohlich C, Denhaerynck K, et al. Prevalence and contributors to fatigue in individuals hospitalized with advanced cancer: a prospective, observational study. Int J Nurs Stud. 2012;49:1146–1154.
92. Annunziata MA, Muzzatti B, Mella S, Bidoli E. Fatigue, quality of life, and mood states during chemotherapy in Italian cancer patients. Tumori. 2013;99:e28–33.
93. Irvine D, Vincent L, Graydon JE, Bubela N, Thompson L. The prevalence and correlates of fatigue in patients receiving treatment with chemotherapy and radiotherapy. A comparison with the fatigue experienced by healthy individuals. Cancer Nurs. 1994;17:367–378.
94. Oh HS, Seo WS. Systematic review and meta-analysis of the correlates of cancer-related fatigue. Worldviews Evid Based Nurs. 2011;8:191–201.
95. Peters MEWJ, Goedendorp MM, Verhagen CAHHVM, Bleijenberg G, van der Graaf WTA. Fatigue and its associated psychosocial factors in cancer patients on active palliative treatment measured over time. Supportive Care in Cancer. 2016;24:1349-1355.
96. Servaes P, Gielissen MF, Verhagen S, Bleijenberg G. The course of severe fatigue in disease-free breast cancer patients: a longitudinal study. Psychooncology. 2006;16:787–795.
97. Lawrence DP, Kupelnick B, Miller K, Devine D, Lau J. Evidence report on the occurrence, assessment, and treatment of fatigue in cancer patients. J Natl Cancer Inst Monogr. 2004:40–50.
98. Quinten C, et al. Patient self-reports of symptoms and clinician ratings as predictors of overall cancer survival. J Natl Cancer Inst. 2011;103:1851–1858.
99. Oldervoll LM, Loge JH, Lydersen S, et al. Physical exercise for cancer patients with advanced disease: a randomized controlled trial. Oncologist. 2011;16:1649–1657.
100. Culos-Reed SN, Carlson LE, Daroux LM, Hately-Aldous S. A pilot study of yoga for breast cancer survivors: physical and psychological benefits. Psycho-Oncology. 2006;15:891–897.

101. Cohen L, Warneke C, Fouladi RT, et al. Psychological adjustment and sleep quality in a randomized trial of the effects of a Tibetan yoga intervention in patients with lymphoma. Cancer. 2004;100:2253–2260.

102. Cramer H, Lauche R, Klose P, et al. Yoga for improving health-related quality of life, mental health and cancer-related symptoms in women diagnosed with breast cancer. Cochrane Database Syst Rev. 2017 Jan 3;1:CD010802.

103. Roth T. Diagnosis and management of insomnia. Clin Cornerstone. 2000;2(5):28-38.

104. Klink M, Stuart F. Quan. Prevalence of Reported Sleep Disturbances in a General Adult Population and their Relationship to Obstructive Airways Diseases. Chest, Volume 91, Issue 4, April 1987, Pages 540–546.

105. Grandner MA, Martin JL, Patel NP, et al. Age and Sleep Disturbances Among American Men And Women: Data From the U.S. Behavioral Risk Factor Surveillance System. Sleep. 2012;35(3):395-406.

106. Grunstein R. Insomnia. Diagnosis and management. Aust Fam Physician. 2002 Nov;31(11):995-1000.

107. Bloom HG, Ahmed I, Alessi CA, Ancoli-Israel S, Buysse DJ, Kryger MH, et al. Evidence-based recommendations for the assessment and maintenance of sleep disorders in older adults. JAGS. 2009; 57:761–89.

108. Stewart R, Besset A, Bebbington P, et al. Insomnia comorbidity and impact and hypnotic use by age group in a national survey population aged 16 to 74 years. Sleep. 2008; 29:1391–1397.

109. Manjunath NK, Telles S. Influence of Yoga and Ayurveda on self-rated sleep in a geriatric population. Indian J Med Res. 2005 May;121(5):683–690.

110. Vadiraja SH, Rao MR, Nagendra RH, et al. Effects of yoga on symptom management in breast cancer patients: A randomized controlled trial. Int J Yoga. 2009;2:73–79.

111. Mustian KM, Sprod LK, Janelsins M, et al. Multicenter, Randomized Controlled Trial of Yoga for Sleep Quality Among Cancer Survivors. Journal of Clinical Oncology. 2013;31(26):3233-3241.

112. who.int/about/mission/en/ (accessed May 24, 2016).

113. Ravens-Sieberer U, Karow A, Barthel D, Klasen F. How to assess quality of life in child and adolescent psychiatry. Dialogues in Clinical Neuroscience. 2014;16(2):147-158.

114. McDowell I. Measures of self-perceived well-being. Journal of Psychosomatic Research. 2010;69(1):69–79.

115. Ware J. E., Kosinski M., Gandek B. SF-36 Health Survey: Manual & Interpretation Guide. Lincoln, RI, USA: QualityMetric; 2000.

116. cdc.gov/hrqol/ (accessed May 24, 2017).

117. Ware JE, Kosinski M, Keller SD. SF-36 Physical and Mental Health Summary Scales: A User's Manual. Boston, MA: The Health Institute, New England Medical Centre, 1994.

118. EuroQol Group . EuroQol: a new facility for the measurement of health-related quality of life. Health Policy, 1990; 16: 199–208.

119. Skevington SM, Mac Arthur P, Somerset M. Developing items for the WHOQOL: a study of contemporary beliefs about quality of life related to health in Britain. British Journal of Health Psychology, 1997; 2: 55–72.

120. Ferrell BR, Dow KH, Grant M. Measurement of the quality of life in cancer survivors. Quality of Life Research. 1995 Dec;4(6):523–531.

121. Conroy T, Marchal F, Blazeby JM. Quality of life in patients with oesophageal and gastric cancer: an overview. Oncology. 2006;70:391–402.

122. Heydarnejad M, Hassanpour DA, Solati DK. Factors affecting quality of life in cancer patients undergoing chemotherapy. African Health Sciences. 2011;11(2):266-270.

123. Soler-Vila H, Kasl SV, Jones BA. Prognostic significance of psychosocial factors in African-American and white breast cancer patients: a population-based study. Cancer. 2003 Sep 15;98(6):1299–1308.

124. Maisey NR, Norman A, Watson M, Allen MJ, Hill ME, Cunningham D. Baseline quality of life predicts survival in patients with advanced colorectal cancer. Eur J Cancer. 2002;38:1351–7.

125. Coates AS, Hurny C, Peterson HF, Bernhard J, Castinglione-Gertsch M, Gelberg D, Goldhirsch A: Quality of life scores predict outcome in metastatic but not early breast cancer. International Breast Cancer Study Group. J Clin Oncol. 2000, 18: 3768-3774.

126. Montazeri A. Quality of life data as prognostic indicators of survival in cancer patients: an overview of the literature from 1982 to 2008. Health and Quality of Life Outcomes. 2009;7:102.

127. Singh P, Chaturvedi A. Complementary and Alternative Medicine in Cancer Pain Management: A Systematic Review. Indian Journal of Palliative Care. 2015;21(1):105-115.

128. Danhauer SC, Tooze JA, Farmer DF, Campbell CR, McQuellon RP, Barrett R, Miller BE. Restorative yoga for women with ovarian or breast cancer: findings from a pilot study. J Soc Integr Oncol. 2008;6(2):47–58.

129. Harder H, Parlour L, Jenkins V. Randomised controlled trials of yoga interventions for women with breast cancer: A systematic literature review. Supportive Care in Cancer. 2012;20:3055–64.

130. Siedentopf F, Utz-Billing I, Gairing S, Schoenegg W, Kentenich H, Kollak I. Yoga for patients with early breast cancer and its impact on quality of life—a randomized controlled trial. Geburtshilfe Frauenheilkd. 2013;73:311-317.

131. Sharma M, Lingam VC, Nahar VK. A systematic review of yoga interventions as integrative treatment in breast cancer. J Cancer Res Clin Oncol. 2016 Dec;142(12):2523-2540.

132. Carlson, Linda E, Michael S, Kamala DP, Eileen G. Mindfulness-based stress reduction in relation to quality of life, mood, symptoms of stress, and immune parameters in breast and prostate cancer outpatients. Psychosom Med. 2003;65:571–81.

133. Fouladbakhsh JM, Davis JE, Yarandi HN. A pilot study of the feasibility and outcomes of yoga for lung cancer survivors. Oncol Nurs Forum. 2014 Mar 1;41(2):162-74.

134. Danhauer SC, Addington EL, Sohl SJ, et al. Review of yoga therapy during cancer treatment. Support Care Cancer. 2017 Jan 7.

Cardiac Rehabilitation

Cardiac rehabilitation programs are complex interventions prescribed in cardiac patients and include health education, advice on cardiovascular risk reduction, increased physical activity and stress management[1-3].

Most patients enter cardiac rehabilitation after a myocardial infarction, acute coronary syndrome[4], coronary artery bypass grafting, percutaneous coronary intervention[5], heart failure[6] or heart or heart/lung transplant[7]. Cardiac rehabilitation is designed to stabilize, slow down or even regress cardiovascular disease[8]. It is effective in reducing major events (revascularization, unstable angina, and heart failure), even up to ten years following an attack[9]. Meta-analytic studies indicate that with rehabilitation, cardiovascular deaths are reduced by about 20% and sudden death by about 37% during the year after an acute myocardial infraction[10]. There is also a reduction in anxiety and depression which are prevalent among cardiac rehabilitation participants[11]. Patients also experience an improved exercise capacity and functionality, and a better quality of life and well being[12-14].

Complementary and alternative medicine modalities have been used for cardiac rehabilitation[15-17]. Yoga has also been suggested for cardiac rehabilitation[18] and has shown clinical effectiveness in this group[19].

Yoga and Cardiac Rehabilitation

In a study of 45 patients referred for cardiac rehabilitation (18 female and 27 male), researchers assigned them into 3 groups (relaxation, meditation and control). At the end of the study, there was a significant reduction in depression, systolic and diastolic blood pressure and heart rate in the meditation group when compared with the control group[20].

In a single blind prospective randomized parallel two-armed active control study, 250 male participants (35–65 years), who had undergone coronary bypass grafting, were recruited. The yoga group were exposed to three modules (of 30 min each): the first module (up to 6th week) included MSRT (Mind Sound Resonance

Technique), breath awareness and DRT (deep relaxation technique), all done in supine posture. Physical postures and pranayama practices were added in the second (6th week to 6th month) and third (6th month to 12th month) yoga module. Non-yogic intervention for the control group was designed to match the duration (30 min), and the level of physical activity as tolerated. At the end of the study, researchers found that the yoga group had significantly better left ventricular ejection fraction, body mass index and blood glucose. They also exhibited a better positive affect. There was a decrease in perceived stress, depression, and negative affect[21].

In a meta-analysis[22], the authors reviewed two studies investigating the benefits of yoga in patients with chronic heart failure. There were a total of 30 yoga and 29 control patients. They found that yoga compared with control had a positive impact on peak oxygen consumption and health related quality of life.

Conclusion

Yoga is a safe alternative to contemporary exercise programs in patients undergoing cardiac rehabilitation, with similar, if not better, evidence based benefits.

References

1. Hotta SS. Cardiac rehabilitation programs. Health Technol Assess Rep. 1991;(3):1-10.
2. Dalal HM, Doherty P, Taylor RS. Cardiac rehabilitation. BMJ. 2015 Sep 29;351:h5000.
3. Balraj S Heran, Jenny MH Chen, Shah Ebrahim, et al. Exercise-based cardiac rehabilitation for coronary heart disease. Cochrane Database Syst Rev. 2011; (7): CD001800.
4. Pashkow FJ. Issues in contemporary cardiac rehabilitation: a historical perspective. J Am Coll Cardiol. 1993 Mar 1;21(3):822-34.
5. Pasquali S.K., Karen P. Alexander, Laura P. Coombs et al. Effect of Cardiac Rehabilitation on Functional Outcomes After Coronary Revascularization. Am Heart J. 2003;145(3).
6. Ades PA, Keteyian SJ, Balady GJ et al. Cardiac rehabilitation exercise and self-care for chronic heart failure. JACC Heart Fail. 2013 Dec;1(6):540-7.
7. Jon A. Kobashigawa, M.D., David A. Leaf, M.D., Nancy Lee, P.T., Michael P. Gleeson, B.S., HongHu Liu, Ph.D., Michele A. Hamilton, M.D., Jaime D. Moriguchi, M.D., Nobuyuki Kawata, M.D., Kim Einhorn, B.S., Elise Herlihy, R.N., and Hillel Laks, M.D. A Controlled Trial of

Exercise Rehabilitation after Heart Transplantation. N Engl J Med 1999; 340:272-277January 28, 1999DOI: 10.1056/NEJM199901283400404.

8. Balady GJ, et al. Referral, enrollment, and delivery of cardiac rehabilitation/secondary prevention programs at clinical centers and beyond: A presidential advisory from the American Heart Association. Circulation. 2011;124:2951–2960.

9. José M Maroto Monteroa, Rosario Artigao Ramíreza, María D Morales Durána, Carmen de Pablo Zarzosaa, Víctor Abrairab. Cardiac Rehabilitation in Patients With Myocardial Infarction: a 10-Year Follow-Up Study. Rev Esp Cardiol. 2005;58:1181-7. - Vol. 58 Num.10.

10. Pashkow FJ. Issues in contemporary cardiac rehabilitation: a historical perspective. J Am Coll Cardiol. 1993 Mar 1;21(3):822-34.

11. Shen BJ, Wachowiak PS, Brooks LG. Psychosocial factors and assessment in cardiac rehabilitation. Eura Medicophys. 2005 Mar;41(1):75-91.

12. Mayou RA1, Gill D, Thompson DR et al. Depression and anxiety as predictors of outcome after myocardial infarction. Psychosom Med. 2000 Mar-Apr;62(2):212-9.

13. Shen BJ, Wachowiak PS, Brooks LG. Psychosocial factors and assessment in cardiac rehabilitation. Eura Medicophys. 2005 Mar;41(1):75-91.

14. McGee HM, Hevey D, Horgan JH. Psychosocial outcome assessments for use in cardiac rehabilitation service evaluation: a 10-year systematic review. Soc Sci Med. 1999 May;48(10):1373-93.

15. Taylor-Piliae RE, Silva E, Sheremeta SP. Tai Chi as an adjunct physical activity for adults aged 45 years and older enrolled in phase III cardiac rehabilitation. European journal of cardiovascular nursing : journal of the Working Group on Cardiovascular Nursing of the European Society of Cardiology. 2012;11(1):34-43. doi:10.1016/j.ejcnurse.2010.11.001.

16. Nieva R, Safavynia SA, Bishop KL, Sperling L. Herbal, Vitamin, and Mineral Supplement Use in Patients Enrolled in a Cardiac Rehabilitation Program. Journal of cardiopulmonary rehabilitation and prevention. 2012;32(5):270-277.

17. Salmoirago-Blotcher E, Wayne P, Bock BC, et al. Design and methods of the Gentle Cardiac Rehabilitation Study – A behavioral study of tai chi exercise for patients not attending cardiac rehabilitation. Contemporary clinical trials. 2015;43:243-251.

18. Telles S, Naveen KV. Yoga for rehabilitation: an overview. Indian J Med Sci. 1997 Apr;51(4):123-7.

19. Raghuram N, Parachuri VR, Swarnagowri MV, et al. Yoga based cardiac rehabilitation after coronary artery bypass surgery: One-year results on LVEF, lipid profile and psychological states – A randomized controlled study. Indian Heart Journal. 2014;66(5):490-502. doi:10.1016/j.ihj.2014.08.007.

20. Delui MH, Yari M, khouyinezhad G, Amini M, Bayazi MH. Comparison of Cardiac Rehabilitation Programs Combined with Relaxation and Meditation Techniques on Reduction of Depression and Anxiety of Cardiovascular Patients. The Open Cardiovascular Medicine Journal. 2013;7:99-103. doi:10.2174/1874192401307010099.

21. Raghuram N, Parachuri VR, Swarnagowri MV, et al. Yoga based cardiac rehabilitation after coronary artery bypass surgery: One-year results on LVEF, lipid profile and psychological states – A randomized

controlled study. Indian Heart Journal. 2014;66(5):490-502. doi:10.1016/j.ihj.2014.08.007.

22. Gomes-Neto M, Rodrigues-Jr ES, Silva-Jr WM, Carvalho VO. Effects of Yoga in Patients with Chronic Heart Failure: A Meta-Analysis. Arquivos Brasileiros de Cardiologia. 2014;103(5):433-439. doi:10.5935/abc.20140149.

Carpal Tunnel Syndrome

Carpal tunnel syndrome (CTS) is a symptomatic compression neuropathy of the median nerve at the level of the wrist[1]. The median nerve gets squeezed at the carpal tunnel which is formed by the carpal bones and by the transverse carpal ligament[2]. Symptoms include pain and tingling in the hand, particularly in the thumb, index, middle finger and the radial side of the ring finger[3]. These symptoms may be relieved by 'flicking' the wrist[4]. Patients may also experience a reduction of the grip strength and function of the affected hand[5]. Causative factors are related to prolonged postures in extremes of wrist flexion or extension, repetitive use of the flexor muscles, and exposure to vibration[6]. Diagnosis is based on symptoms and clinical examination, which also includes two simple tests. Patients on flexing their wrist for 60 seconds experience pain or paresthesia in the distribution of the median nerve. This is the Phalen's test[7]. In the Tinel's test, tapping over the volar surface of the wrist produces paresthesia over the thumb, index, middle finger and the radial side of the ring finger[8]. Nerve conduction studies usually reveal prolonged motor and sensory latencies and reduced sensory and motor conduction velocities of the median nerve[9]. MRI may also provide more specific details of the entrapment[10].

Carpal tunnel syndrome is estimated to occur in 3.8% of the general population[11]. Occupational causes are often responsible – CTS was diagnosed in almost 5 million U.S. workers in 2010[12]. It is often seen in employed adults – according to the Centers for Disease Control and Prevention (CDC). In 2010, it affected an estimated 3.1% of employed adults aged 18–64 years in the previous 12 months[13]. According to the US Dept. of Labor, it was responsible for more days off work, than any other non-fatal injury[14]. It is more common in women[15]. Systemic conditions often associated with CTS include rheumatoid arthritis, hypothyroidism, diabetes mellitus, acromegaly, gout, and pregnancy[16].

In mild to moderate CTS, non-surgical treatment may be tried - mainly splinting (usually night time immobilization of the wrist in a neutral position for six or more weeks) and oral prednisone or intercarpal injections of steroids[17]. In patients with severe disease, surgical treatment may be considered. It consists of reducing the pressure on the median nerve by dividing the transverse carpal ligament and thereby increasing the space in the carpal tunnel[18]. However, these treatment modalities may only provide short term relief in some patients[19].

Yoga and Carpel Tunnel Syndrome

Yoga has been suggested as one form of conservative treatment for CTS[20].

In a study of 42 patients having pain from carpal tunnel syndrome, patients were assigned to either an Iyengar-based Hatha yoga protocol or a control treatment (wrist splint). At the end of eight weeks, the yoga group patients experienced significant reductions in pain (decreased from 5.0 to 2.9 mm; P = .02). There was also an improvement in the grip strength (increased from 162 to 187 mm Hg; P = .009). Phalen's sign also improved (12 improved vs 2 in control group; P = .008) in the yoga group[21].

O'Connor and associates mention one trial involving 51 people with CTS, where yoga significantly reduced pain after eight weeks (WMD -1.40; 95% CI -2.73 to -0.07) compared with wrist splinting[22].

There is limited evidence of the efficacy of yoga in the long-term treatment of carpel tunnel syndrome[23].

Conclusion

Yoga may be beneficial in the short term in patients with CTS, especially for reduction of pain.

References

1. Ibrahim I, Khan WS, Goddard N, Smitham P. Carpal tunnel syndrome: a review of the recent literature. Open Orthop J. 2012;6:69–76.
2. Alfonso C, Jann S, Massa R, Torreggiani A. Diagnosis treatment and follow-up of the carpal tunnel syndrome: a review. Neurolog Sci. 2010;31(3):243–52.
3. Solomon L, Warwick D, Nayagam S. Apley's concise system of orthopaedics and fractures. NY: Oxford University Press; 2005.
4. Krendel DA, Jobsis M, Gaskell PC, Jr, Sanders DB. The flick sign in carpal tunnel syndrome. J Neurol Neurosurg Psychiatr. 1986;49(2): 220–1.

5. Zyluk A, Kosovets L. An assessment of the sympathetic function within the hand in patients with carpal tunnel syndrome. J Hand Surg Eur Vol. 2010;35(5):402–8.

6. Martin S. Carpal tunnel syndrome a job-related risk. Am Pharmacy. 1991;31(8):21–4.

7. Phalen GS. The carpal tunnel syndrome seventeen years: experience in diagnosis and treatment of six hundred fifty-four hands. J Bone Joint Surg. 1966;48A:211–28.

8. Almasi-Doghaee M, Boostani R, Saeedi M, Ebrahimzadeh S, Moghadam-Ahmadi A, Saeedi-Borujeni MJ. Carpal compression, Phalen's and Tinel's test: Which one is more suitable for carpal tunnel syndrome? Iranian Journal of Neurology. 2016;15(3):173-174.

9. LeBlanc KE, Cestia W. Carpal tunnel syndrome. Am Fam Physician. 2011;83:952–958.

10. Khalil C, Hancart C, Le Thuc V, Chantelot C, Chechin D, Cotten A. Diffusion tensor imaging and tractography of the median nerve in carpal tunnel syndrome: preliminary results. Eur Radiol. 2008;18:2283–2291.

11. Uchiyama S, Itsubo T, Nakamura K, Kato H, Yasutomi T, Momose T. Current concepts of carpal tunnel syndrome: pathophysiology, treatment, and evaluation. J Orthop Sci. 2010;15:1–13.

12. Luckhaupt SE, Dahlhamer JM, Ward BW, Sweeney MH, Sestito JP, Calvert GM. Prevalence and work-relatedness of carpal tunnel syndrome in the working population, United States, 2010 National Health Interview Survey. Am J Ind Med. 2013 Jun;56(6):615-24. doi: 10.1002/ajim.22048. Epub 2012 Apr 11.

13. cdc.gov/mmwr/preview/mmwrhtml/mm6049a4.htm - accessed 12/30/17.

14. bls.gov/opub/ted/2001/apr/wk1/art01.htm - accessed 12/30/17.

15. Ibrahim I, Khan WS, Goddard N, Smitham P. Carpal tunnel syndrome: a review of the recent literature. Open Orthop J. 2012;6:69–76.

16. Practice parameter for carpal tunnel syndrome [summary statement]. Report of the Quality Standards Subcommittee of the American Academy of Neurology. Neurology. 1993;43:2406–2409.

17. Shi Q, MacDermid JC. Is surgical intervention more effective than non-surgical treatment for carpal tunnel syndrome? A systematic review. J Orthop Surg Res. 2011;6:17.

18. Aroori S, Spence RA. Carpal tunnel syndrome. Ulster Med J. 2008;77:6–17.

19. Gerritsen AA, de Vet HC, Scholten RJ, van Tulder MW, Bouter LM. Enabling meta-analysis in systematic reviews on carpal tunnel syndrome. J. Hand Surg. Am. 2002;27:828–832.

20. Bland JDP. Carpal tunnel syndrome. BMJ□: British Medical Journal. 2007;335(7615):343-346. doi:10.1136/bmj.39282.623553.AD.

21. Garfinkel MS, Singhal A, Katz WA, Allan DA, Reshetar R, Schumacher HR., Jr Yoga-based intervention for carpal tunnel syndrome: a randomized trial. JAMA. 1998;280:1601–3.

22. O'Connor D, Marshall S, Massy-Westropp N. Non-surgical treatment (other than steroid injection) for carpal tunnel syndrome. Cochrane Database Syst Rev. 2003;(1):CD003219.

23. Piazzini DB, Aprile I, Ferrara PE, Bertolini C, Tonali P, Maggi L, Rabini A, Piantelli S, Padua L. A systematic review of conservative treatment of carpal tunnel syndrome. Clin Rehabil. 2007 Apr;21(4):299-314.

Cerebral Palsy

Cerebral Palsy is a leading cause of motor disability in children[1]. It is estimated that it affects two to three of every 1000 live births in the United States[2,3]. It has a worldwide prevalence of one to five in every 1000 live births[4]. Children suffering from cerebral palsy exhibit abnormal muscle tone or posture, delayed motor milestones, and gait abnormalities[5]. Although the damage occurs in the developing brain during the fetus or infant stage[6], the musculo-skeletal manifestations continue to worsen as the child grows, and the functional impairment gets progressively poor[7]. Diagnosis is based on history, symptoms and signs. MRI is the gold standard in its diagnosis and will identify neural injury in these patients[8]. Treatment is aimed at giving physical therapy and adaptive equipment. Patients may also require drug therapy and surgical interventions[9]. Complementary and alternative medicine modalities have been suggested[10,11]. Yoga is also being studied in this population.

Yoga and Cerebral Palsy

A study on the benefit of mindfulness movement program based on hatha yoga in patients with cerebral palsy is underway and the results are awaited[12].

In a study of 43 health care providers of patients with neurological problems, including cerebral palsy, two groups, (yoga n=20 and control group n=23) were evaluated at the end of one month. The researchers noted a significant decrease in anxiety and depression scores in the yoga group. They also reported an improved quality-of-life in the yoga group[13].

Conclusion

Evidence based data on the benefit of yoga in cerebral palsy patients is awaited.

References

1. Capute and Accardo's Neurodevelopmental Disabilities in Infancy and Childhood, Third Edition. Edited by Pasquale J. Accardo, MD. 2008, Paul H. Brookes Publishing Co, Baltimore, MD. p17.

2. Yeargin-Allsopp M, Braun KVN, Doernberg NS, Benedict RE, Kirby RS, Durkin MS. Prevalence of cerebral palsy in 8-year-old children in three areas of the United States in 2002: a multisite collaboration. Pediatrics. 2008;121(3):547–554.
3. Oskoui M., Coutinho F., Dykeman J., Jetté N., Pringsheim T. An update on the prevalence of cerebral palsy: a systematic review and meta-analysis. Dev Med Child Neurol. 2013 Jun;55(6):509-19. doi: 10.1111/dmcn.12080. Epub 2013 Jan 24.
4. Vincer MJ, Allen AC, Joseph KS, Stinson DA, Scott H, Wood E. Increasing prevalence of cerebral palsy among very preterm infants: a population-based study. Pediatrics. Pediatrics. 2006 Dec;118(6): e1621-6. Epub 2006 Oct 30.
5. Wu Y. W., Croen L. A., Shah S. J., Newman T. B., Najjar D. V. (2006). Cerebral palsy in a term population: risk factors and neuroimaging findings. Pediatrics 118 690–697. 10.1542/peds.2006-0278.
6. Rosenbaum P., Paneth N., Leviton A., Goldstein M., Damiano D., Dan B., et al. (2007). A report: the definition and classification of cerebral palsy April 2006. Dev. Med. Child Neurol. 49 8–14. 10.1111/j.1469-8749.2007.tb12610.x.
7. Sanger T. D. (2015). Movement disorders in cerebral palsy. J. Pediatr. Neurol. 13 198–207.
8. Fiori S., Guzzetta A., Pannek K., Ware R. S., Rossi G., Klingels K., et al. (2015). Validity of semi-quantitative scale for brain MRI in unilateral cerebral palsy due to periventricular white matter lesions: relationship with hand sensorimotor function and structural connectivity. Neuroimage 8 104–109. 10.1016/j.nicl.2015.04.005.
9. http://www.cerebralpalsy.org/about-cerebral-palsy/treatment - accessed 1/28/17
10. Oppenheim WL. Complementary and alternative methods in cerebral palsy. Dev Med Child Neurol. 2009 Oct;51 Suppl 4:122-9. doi: 10.1111/j.1469-8749.2009.03424.x.
11. Shailaja U, Rao PN, Debnath P, Adhikari A. Exploratory study on the ayurvedic therapeutic management of cerebral palsy in children at a tertiary care hospital of karnataka, India. J Tradit Complement Med. 2014 Jan;4(1):49-55. doi: 10.4103/2225-4110.124345.
12. Catherine Mak, Koa Whittingham, Ross Cunnington, Roslyn N Boyd. MiYoga: a randomised controlled trial of a mindfulness movement programme based on hatha yoga principles for children with cerebral palsy: a study protocol. BMJ Open. 2017; 7(7): e015191. Published online 2017 Jul 10. doi: 10.1136/bmjopen-2016-015191.
13. P. Umadevi, Ramachandra, S. Varambally, M. Philip, B. N. Gangadhar. Effect of yoga therapy on anxiety and depressive symptoms and quality-of-life among caregivers of in-patients with neurological disorders at a tertiary care center in India: A randomized controlled trial. Indian J Psychiatry. 2013 Jul; 55(Suppl 3): S385–S389. doi: 10.4103/0019-5545.11630.

Chronic Fatigue Syndrome

Chronic fatigue syndrome (CFS) is characterized by unexplained intense fatigue (new in onset) of more than six months duration as well as presence of at least four of the following physical symptoms: post exertional malaise of more than 24 hours; unrefreshing sleep, impaired memory or concentration, muscle pain, polyarthralgia, tender lymph nodes or new headaches[1]. It is often associated with other symptoms, such as anxiety, depression and cognitive dysfunction[2]. Although various theories have been advanced[3], the etiology remains unclear. The fatigue is usually intense and permanent. Its prevalence ranges from 0.007% to 2.5% in the general population[4]. Diagnosis is based on the clinical history and symptoms and there is no diagnostic test or markers establishing the presence of this disease. There are no pharmacologic agents for this disease. Treatment consists of graded exercise therapy and cognitive behavioral therapy[5]. Yoga has been recently tried in these patients[6].

Yoga and Chronic Fatigue Syndrome

In a trial of 30 patients with CFS, without satisfactory improvement after receiving conventional therapy for at least six months, the participants were randomly divided into two groups. The control group of 15 participants was given conventional therapy while the yoga group of 15 participants was continued on conventional therapy combined with isometric yoga. Yoga practice consisted of biweekly, 20-minute sessions with a yoga instructor and daily in-home sessions for approximately two months. Fatigue was determined by Profile of Mood Status questionnaire to evaluate short term benefits and by Chalder's Fatigue Scale questionnaire to evaluate long term benefits. The yoga group showed an improvement with scores for both questionnaires decreasing significantly when compared to that reported by the control group[7]. These findings have been confirmed recently[8].

Conclusion

Preliminary data suggest beneficial effects of yoga practice in patients with chronic fatigue syndrome.

References

1. Fukuda K, Straus SE, Hickie I, Sharpe MC, Dobbins JG, Komaroff A; International Chronic Fatigue Syndrome Study Group. The chronic fatigue syndrome: a comprehensive approach to its definition and study. Ann Intern Med. 1994;121(12):953–959.
2. Wyller VB. The chronic fatigue syndrome--an update. Acta Neurol Scand Suppl. 2007;187:7–14. doi: 10.1111/j.1600-0404.2007.00840.x. Review.
3. Bassi N, Amital D, Amital H, Doria A, Shoenfeld Y. Chronic fatigue syndrome: characteristics and possible causes for its pathogenesis. Isr Med Assoc J. 2008;10:79–82.
4. Jason LA, Richman JA, Rademaker AW, Jordan KM, Plioplys AV, Taylor RR, Mc Cready W, Huang CF, Plioplys S. A community based study of chronic fatigue syndrome. Arch Intern Med. 1999;159:2129–2137. doi: 10.1001/archinte.159.18.2129.
5. Whiting P, Bagnall A, Sowden A. Interventions for the treatment and management of chronic fatigue syndrome: a systematic review. JAMA. 2001;286:1360–8. doi: 10.1001/jama.286.11.1360.
6. Yadav RK, Sarvottam K, Magan D, Yadav R. A two-year follow-up case of chronic fatigue syndrome: substantial improvement in personality following a yoga-based lifestyle intervention. J Altern Complement Med. 2015 Apr;21(4):246-9. doi: 10.1089/acm.2014.0055. Epub 2015 Mar 31.
7. Oka T, Tanahashi T, Chijiwa T, Lkhagvasuren B, Sudo N, Oka K. Isometric yoga improves the fatigue and pain of patients with chronic fatigue syndrome who are resistant to conventional therapy: a randomized, controlled trial. Biopsychosocial Medicine. 2014;8:27. doi:10.1186/s13030-014-0027-8.
8. Oka T, Wakita H, Kimura K. Development of a recumbent isometric yoga program for patients with severe chronic fatigue syndrome/myalgic encephalomyelitis: A pilot study to assess feasibility and efficacy. Biopsychosoc Med. 2017 Mar 3;11:5. doi: 10.1186/s13030-017-0090-z. eCollection 2017.

Chronic Kidney Disease

It is estimated that during the years 1999-2004, the prevalence of chronic kidney disease (CKD) in the United States was 13.1%[1]. Globally, it affects between 10% and 16% of all adults[2]. Diabetes mellitus is the most common cause of kidney failure in the United States, accounting for about 44% of new cased[3]. Hypertension is also a major cause of CKD[4,5]. Other causes of CKD include glomerulonephritis and polycystic kidney diseases. The presence of CKD increases the risks of several other diseases, especially, cardiovascular disease[6]. The co-existence of cardiovascular disease in these patients increases the morbidity and mortality[7]. Treatment for end stage renal disease is dialysis or transplantation. Mortality per year can be as high as 20% in patients on dialysis[8]. Kidney transplant is often limited by organ shortage and 13 people die each day while waiting for a life-saving kidney transplant[9]. Complementary and alternative medicine use is common in CKD patients[10,11].

Yoga and Chronic Kidney Disease

In a study reported recently[12], fifty-four patients with CKD were divided into two groups: a yoga group (conventional treatment plus yoga) and a control group (conventional treatment alone). Patients in the yoga group performed specific yogic asanas for at least 5 days a week for 40–60 min a day. Fifty patients, 25 in each group, completed 6 months of monitoring. At the end of the study, the yoga group demonstrated a significant reduction in systolic and diastolic blood pressure, significant reduction in blood urea and serum creatinine levels, and significant improvement in physical and psychological domain of the World Health Organization quality of life (QOL). On the other hand, the control group worsened, exhibiting a rise in blood pressure and deterioration of renal function. Their QOL scores also deteriorated.

Conclusion

Yoga practice appears to delay the need for dialysis in CKD patients, in one study.

References

1. Coresh J, Selvin E, Stevens LA, Manzi J, Kusek JW, Eggers P, Van Lente F, Levey AS. Prevalence of chronic kidney disease in the United States. JAMA. 2007;298:2038–2047.
2. Mills KT, Xu Y, Zhang W, Bundy JD, Chen CS, Kelly TN, Chen J, He J. A systematic analysis of worldwide population-based data on the global burden of chronic kidney disease in 2010. Kidney Int. 2015;88(5):950–957. doi: 10.1038/ki.2015.230.
3. https://www.kidney.org/news/newsroom/factsheets/Diabetes-And-CKD - accessed 2/1/18 - accessed 11/3/17.
4. Klag MJ, Whelton PK, Randall BL, et al. Blood pressure and end-stage renal disease in men. N Engl J Med. 1996;334(1):13–18.
5. Klag MJ, Whelton PK, Randall BL, et al. Blood pressure and end-stage renal disease in men. N Engl J Med. 1996;334(1):13–18.
6. Gargiulo R, Suhail F, Lerma EV. Cardiovascular disease and chronic kidney disease. Dis Mon. 2015;61:403–413.
7. Herzog CA, et al. Cardiovascular disease in chronic kidney disease. A clinical update from Kidney Disease: Improving Global Outcomes (KDIGO) Kidney international. 2011;80:572–586.
8. Kovesdy CP, et al. Outcomes associated with microalbuminuria: effect modification by chronic kidney disease. Journal of the American College of Cardiology. 2013;61:1626–1633.
9. http://optn.transplant.hrsa.gov/ - accessed 2/1/18.
10. Spanner ED, Duncan AM. Prevalence of dietary supplement use in adults with chronic renal insufficiency. J Ren Nutr. 2005 Apr; 15(2):204-10.
11. Arjuna Rao AS, Phaneendra D, Pavani ChD, Soundararajan P, Rani NV, Thennarasu P, Kannan G. Usage of complementary and alternative medicine among patients with chronic kidney disease on maintenance hemodialysis. J Pharm Bioallied Sci. 2016 Jan-Mar;8(1):52-7. doi: 10.4103/0975-7406.171692.
12. Rajendra Kumar Pandey, Tung Vir Singh Arya, Amit Kumar, Ashish Yadav. Effects of 6 months yoga program on renal functions and quality of life in patients suffering from chronic kidney disease. Int J Yoga. 2017 Jan-Apr; 10(1): 3–8. doi: 10.4103/0973-6131.186158.

COPD

Chronic obstructive pulmonary disease (COPD) is a major cause of morbidity and mortality. It poses a major public health problem worldwide[1]. According to the latest World Health Organization (WHO) estimates, there were 64 million people with COPD and 3 million people died of COPD in 2004. The number of deaths from COPD are on the rise in the US[2]. WHO predicts that COPD will become the third leading cause of death worldwide by 2030[3].

More than 90% of COPD deaths occur in low- and middle-income countries. Its social burden is expected to rank fifth in the world by 2020[4]. COPD is characterized by irreversible airflow obstruction, a gradual decline in lung function, loss of lung tissue, reduced quality of life, and a high rate of mortality[5]. The Global Initiative for Chronic Obstructive Lung Disease (GOLD) management aims at a reduction in symptoms, complications, and exacerbations, improved exercise tolerance, better health status, and reduced mortality[6]. Some of these goals can be achieved by initiating breathing exercises in these patients[7]. Although not curable, a host of pharmacological and non-pharmacological modalities are available to help control symptoms and improve the quality of life for these patients. Treatment consists of long-acting bronchodilators, inhaled corticosteroids as a combination therapy. Oral PED4 inhibitors are also used as an add on therapy after inhaled corticosteroids. Non-pharmacological treatment includes pulmonary rehabilitation, exercise, vaccination against influenza (all COPD patients) and pneumococcus (all COPD patients older than 65 or with other cardiopulmonary disease) and palliative care. Oral opioids are sometimes used in severe COPD symptoms refractory to medical therapy. Yoga is emerging as a valuable complementary modality, in COPD[8,9].

Yoga and COPD

In a study of 33 COPD patients, conventional treatment was continued while they were trained to do breathing exercises, meditation, and yoga postures for 1 hour, thrice a week for 6 weeks. At the end of the study, Fulambarkar and associates noted statistically significant improvements in vital capacity, maximal inspiratory pressure and maximal expiratory pressure in these patients[10].

In a systemic review and meta-analysis of five randomized controlled trials involving 233 patients, investigators reached the conclusion that yoga training resulted in a significantly improved forced expiratory volume in the first second (FEV1), FEV1% predicted, and the distance achieved on the six-minute walk test[11].

Depression and anxiety are common in patients with COPD[12,13]. Improvement in these co-morbidities helps improve the quality of life in these patients[14]. Yoga helps reduce depression and anxiety in COPD patients. In a randomized trial involving 81 coal miners (aged 36-60 years), participants were divided into two study arms (yoga and control). Conventional care was carried on in both groups while the treatment group also participated in a yoga program for 12 weeks. Using COPD Assessment Test, Beck Depression Inventory and State and Trait Anxiety Inventory at the beginning and the end of the interventions, the researchers reported greater improvement in the physical and mental health status (depression and anxiety) in the yoga group[15].

In another study, 29 stable patients with COPD were randomized to a 12-week yoga program or usual-care control. At the end of the study, yoga participants showed an improved six-minute walk distance, functional performance and health related quality of life[16].

In a study of 60 patients with COPD, randomly divided into 2 groups – one underwent yoga exercises and the other group underwent pulmonary rehabilitation. The interventions were for one hour twice a week for the first 4 weeks. During the next 8 weeks, supervised sessions were given fortnightly and the remaining sessions were done by the patients at home. Assessments at baseline and at the end of 12 weeks included measurement of lung functions and dyspnea assessment[17]. The improvements were similar in both groups. The authors concluded that yoga practice was as good as pulmonary rehabilitation in these patients[18].

Yoga is well tolerated by COPD patients[19].

Conclusion

Yoga practice is an efficacious complimentary modality for the long-term management of COPD.

References

1. Murray CJ, Lopez AD. Mortality by cause for eight regions of the world: Global burden of disease study. Lancet. 1997;349: 1269–76.
2. Jiemin Ma, Elizabeth M. Ward, Rebecca L. Siegel, et al. Temporal Trends in Mortality in the United States, 1969-2013. JAMA. 2015;314(16):1731-1739.
3. WHO, 2004: http://www.who.int/respiratory/copd/en/; (accessed October 2015).
4. Viegi G, Pistelli F, Sherrill DL, et al. Definition, epidemiology and natural history of COPD. Eur Respir J 2007;30: 993-1013.;   Murray CJ, Lopez AD. Mortality by cause for eight regions of the world: Global burden of disease study. Lancet. 1997;349: 1269–76.
5. National Institutes of Health; 2006. Global initiative for chronic obstructive lung disease, Global strategy for the diagnosis, management and prevention of COPD: NHLBI/WHO workshop report; pp. 5–6.
6. Vestbo J, Hurd SS, Agusti AG, et al. Global strategy for the diagnosis, management, and prevention of chronic obstructive pulmonary disease: GOLD executive summary. Am J Respir Crit Care Med 2013; 187:347-65.
7. Holland AE, Hill CJ, Jones AY, McDonald CF. Breathing exercises for chronic obstructive pulmonary disease. Cochrane Database Syst Rev. 2012 Oct 17;10:CD008250.
8. DorAnne Donesky-Cuenco, Huong Q. Nguyen, Steven Paul, et al. Yoga Therapy Decreases Dyspnea-Related Distress and Improves Functional Performance in People with Chronic Obstructive Pulmonary Disease: A Pilot Study. J Altern Complement Med. 2009 Mar; 15(3): 225–234.
9. Liu XC, Pan L, Hu Q, et al. Effects of yoga training in patients with chronic obstructive pulmonary disease: a systematic review and meta-analysis. J Thorac Dis. 2014 Jun;6(6):795-802.
10. Fulambarker A, Farooki B, Kheir F, Copur AS, Srinivasan L, Schultz S. Effect of yoga in chronic obstructive pulmonary disease. Am J Ther. 2012 Mar;19(2):96-100. doi: 10.1097/MJT.0b013e3181f2ab86.
11. Liu X-C, Pan L, Hu Q, Dong W-P, Yan J-H, Dong L. Effects of yoga training in patients with chronic obstructive pulmonary disease: a systematic review and meta-analysis. Journal of Thoracic Disease. 2014;6(6):795-802. doi:10.3978/j.issn.2072-1439.2014.06.05.
12. Panagioti M, Scott C, Blakemore A, Coventry PA. Overview of the prevalence, impact, and management of depression and anxiety in chronic obstructive pulmonary disease. Int J Chron Obstruct Pulmon Dis. 2014;9:1289–306.

13. Pumar MI, Gray CR, Walsh JR, Yang IA, Rolls TA, Ward DL. Anxiety and depression—Important psychological comorbidities of COPD. Journal of Thoracic Disease. 2014;6(11):1615-1631. doi:10.3978/j.issn.2072-1439.2014.09.28.
14. Blakemore A, Dickens C, Guthrie E, et al. Depression and anxiety predict health-related quality of life in chronic obstructive pulmonary disease: systematic review and meta-analysis. Int J Chron Obstruct Pulmon Dis. 2014;9:501–512.
15. Ranjita R, Badhai S, Hankey A, Nagendra HR. A randomized controlled study on assessment of health status, depression, and anxiety in coal miners with chronic obstructive pulmonary disease following yoga training. International Journal of Yoga. 2016;9(2):137-144. doi:10.4103/0973-6131.183714.
16. Donesky-Cuenco D, Nguyen HQ, Paul S, Carrieri-Kohlman V. Yoga Therapy Decreases Dyspnea-Related Distress and Improves Functional Performance in People with Chronic Obstructive Pulmonary Disease: A Pilot Study. Journal of Alternative and Complementary Medicine. 2009;15(3):225-234. doi:10.1089/acm.2008.0389.
17. Borg scale, VAS, six-minute walk test), quality of life and serum inflammatory markers (CRP and Il-6).
18. Guleria R, et al "Yoga is as effective as standard pulmonary rehabilitation in improving dyspnea, inflammatory markers, and quality of life in patients with COPD" Chest 2015; DOI: 10.1378/chest.2266469.
19. Pomidori L, Campigotto F, Amatya TM, et al. Efficacy and tolerability of yoga breathing in patients with chronic obstructive pulmonary disease: a pilot study. J Cardiopulm Rehabil Prev. 2009 Mar-Apr;29(2):133-7.

Coronary Artery Disease

Cardiovascular disease is the leading cause of death in the world. It is responsible for 31% of all global deaths[1]. It is estimated that in the year 2030, cardiovascular diseases will be responsible for 23.6 million deaths worldwide[2,3]. Cardiovascular disease is also the leading cause of death in the USA[4].

In the USA, coronary artery disease (CAD) is the most common form of cardiovascular disease.[5] It caused approximately 1 of every 6 deaths in the United States in 2010[6]. According to this report, one American has a coronary event approximately every 34 seconds and one American will die from it approximately every 1 minute 23 seconds[6]. Coronary artery disease is responsible for about 370,000 deaths annually in the United States[7]. More than 95 percent of all coronary artery disease is due to atherosclerosis[8]. Atherosclerosis is a chronic inflammatory disease[9], and causes plaque formation inside the coronary arteries. Cardiovascular risk factors aggravate the inflammation, and thus contribute to the pathogenesis of coronary artery disease[10].

The major risk factors include hypertension, cigarette smoking, diabetes mellitus or elevated glucose levels, abnormal cholesterol levels, inactivity and obesity/overweight[11,12]. Genetics and some other still unidentified risk factors also play a role[13].

Patients with CAD can present with stable angina pectoris, unstable angina pectoris, or a myocardial infarction[14]. Sudden death may also be the first manifestation of coronary artery disease[15]. Novel biomarkers[16] and advanced invasive[17] and non-invasive[18] techniques have greatly allowed accurate diagnosis of CAD. Treatment is aimed at improving lifestyle[19], medications, stenting and bypass surgery[20,21].

Cardiac rehabilitation also has been beneficial in its management[22-24]. Complementary and alternative therapies are popular[25-27], and yoga appears appealing[28].

Yoga and Coronary Artery Disease

Yoga and yogic lifestyle have been shown to reduce most risk factors for coronary artery disease. These include reductions in high blood pressure, obesity, hypercholesterolemia, diabetes mellitus, smoking and inactivity[29]. Except for hypercholesterolemia and inactivity, the other risk factors are individually discussed under their own headings in this book. A brief mention is made here.

Yoga practice has been consistently associated with a decrease in blood pressure. In a meta-analytic review of 17 studies (22 trials), yoga was associated with a small but significant decline in both systolic and diastolic blood pressure (−4.17 and −3.26 mmHg respectively)[30]. Several other analyses have reached similar conclusions[31-33].

Yogic lifestyle also results in weight loss. In a coronary artery disease study involving 42 men with angiographically proven CAD, a yoga (along with diet control, control of other risk factors and moderate aerobic exercise) intervention group was compared with a control group. Interventions for one year in 21 men in the yoga group resulted in a decrease in body weight, when compared to the 21 men in the control group[34]. Several other studies have confirmed weight loss associated with yoga practice[35-38].

Many studies have reported that yoga improves lipid profiles in not only healthy individuals[39,40], but also in hypertensive patients[41]. It also improves the lipid profiles in people at risk for coronary artery disease[42] and in those with diabetes mellitus[43]. In a meta-analysis, Innes and group reported that in 8 non-randomized control trials (N = 737 participants) yoga participants registered significant improvements in lipid profiles. These included reductions in levels of total cholesterol, low-density lipoprotein cholesterol, very low-density lipoprotein cholesterol, and triglycerides, and increases in high-density lipoprotein cholesterol, relative to standard care[44].

Yoga may play a complementary role in reducing the risks associated with prediabetes[45], and established diabetes[46]. Yoga is beneficial even if the diabetes is poorly controlled[47].

Yoga practice in several studies has helped patients stop smoking[48]. In a review of four studies, Todd and associates found that the practice of yoga helped smokers quit. The yoga practitioners had increased desire and motivation to quit smoking. They had fewer urges to smoke and reduced temptations to smoke[50]. Yogic breathing has also shown to reduce the craving for cigarettes[50]. In a review of 19 randomized controlled trials, Klinsophon and group concluded that yoga when combined with cognitive-behavioral therapy demonstrated a positive effect on smoking cessation[51].

Physical inactivity has deleterious health effects, comparable to smoking and obesity[52]. with a major percentage developing cardiovascular diseases[53.] Yoga is a low intensity and low impact exercise[54]. Yoga, using the body's own weight and the natural gravity, puts the body through a wide range of motion[55,56]. Yoga routines, despite their low energy expenditure[56], improve many cardiorespiratory fitness parameters, and could be used in place of other aerobic activities recommended by current guidelines for cardiovascular disease prevention[57].

Besides the reduction in the severity of risk factors for CAD, yoga practice also demonstrates other beneficial effects.

Several studies have also reported an improved heart rate variability due to increased parasympathetic and reduced sympathetic activity in the yoga patients. There are also reductions in inflammatory biomarkers such as C-reactive protein (CRP), interleukin IL-6 and tumor necrosis factor TNF-a[58,59]. Biomarkers of stress, namely, cortisol and beta-endorphin are also reduced[60,61]. These positive modulations suggest a potential role in primary prevention of coronary artery disease. Its role is secondary prevention has also been suggested[62].

Studies have also shown an improvement in several pulmonary parameters in patients with coronary artery disease with pranayama practice[63]. In a study of 80 patients with coronary artery disease, yoga practice (40 patients) resulted in statistically significant improvements in slow vital capacity, forced vital capacity, peak expiratory flow rate, maximum voluntary ventilation, and diffusion factor/ transfer factor of lung for carbon monoxide after 3 months of yoga regimen, when compared to patients in the usual care group (also 40 patients)[64].

Studies have also reported a regression in coronary atherosclerosis with yoga and yogic lifestyle intervention[34]. In another study of coronary artery disease patients (71 patients in study group and 42 patients in control group), the study group was given a family based yoga program which included, control of risk factors, dietary modifications and stress management for a period of one year. At the end of the study, the yoga group showed statistical significant reductions in serum total cholesterol and serum low density lipoprotein cholesterol. These patients also demonstrated regression of disease, arrest of progression and limited progression in many patients in the yoga group, when compared to the controls[65].

Depression is pathological in patients with coronary artery disease[66], and yogic techniques have demonstrated effectiveness in improving mood in these patients[67]. Yoga practice also improves functionality as well as mentation in patients following a heart attack[68,69].

Conclusion

Yoga and yogic lifestyle have a real potential of preventing, controlling the progression of, or even regressing coronary artery disease.

References

1. http://www.who.int/mediacentre/factsheets/fs317/en/- accessed 1/12/18
2. Dalen JE, Alpert JS, Goldberg RJ, Weinstein RS. The epidemic of the 20(th) century: coronary heart disease. Am J Med. 2014;127:807–812.
3. Wong ND. Epidemiological studies of CHD and the evolution of preventive cardiology. Nat Rev Cardiol. 2014;11:276–289.
4. https://www.cdc.gov/heartdisease/facts.htm - accesed 1/16/18.
5. CDC, NCHS. Underlying Cause of Death 1999-2013 on CDC WONDER Online Database, released 2015. Data are from the Multiple Cause of Death Files, 1999-2013, as compiled from data provided by the 57 vital statistics jurisdictions through the Vital Statistics Cooperative Program. Accessed Feb. 3, 2015.
6. Go AS, Mozaffarian D, Roger VL, Benjamin EJ, Berry JD, Blaha MJ, Dai S, Ford ES, Fox CS, Franco S, et al. Heart disease and stroke statistics-

-2014 update: a report from the American Heart Association. Circulation. 2014;129: e28–e292.

7. CDC, NCHS. Underlying Cause of Death 1999-2013 on CDC WONDER Online Database, released 2015. Data are from the Multiple Cause of Death Files, 1999-2013, as compiled from data provided by the 57 vital statistics jurisdictions through the Vital Statistics Cooperative Program. Accessed October 21, 2015.CDC, 2015.

8. Mallika V, Goswami B, Rajappa M. Atherosclerosis pathophysiology and the role of novel risk factors: a clinicobiochemical perspective. Angiology 2007;58:513-22.

9. Ross R. Atherosclerosis--an inflammatory disease. N Engl J Med. 1999;340(2):115–126.

10. Mallika V, Goswami B, Rajappa M. Atherosclerosis pathophysiology and the role of novel risk factors: a clinicobiochemical perspective. Angiology 2007;58:513-22.

11. Wilson PW, et al. Prediction of coronary heart disease using risk factor categories. Circulation. 1998;97:1837–1847.

12. Berenson GS, Srinivasan SR, Bao W, Newman WP, 3rd, Tracy RE, Wattigney WA. Association between multiple cardiovascular risk factors and atherosclerosis in children and young adults. The Bogalusa Heart Study. N Engl J Med. 1998;338:1650–1656.

13. Winkelmann BR, Hager J. Genetic variation in coronary heart disease and myocardial infarction: methodological overview and clinical evidence. Pharmacogenomics. 2000 Feb;1(1):73-94.

14. https://www.nhlbi.nih.gov/health-topics/coronary-heart-disease - accessed 1/7/18.

15. Douglas P. Zipes, Hein J. J. Wellens. Sudden Cardiac Death. Circulation. 1998;98:2334-2351.

16. Infante T, Forte E, Schiano C, et al. An integrated approach to coronary heart disease diagnosis and clinical management. American Journal of Translational Research. 2017;9(7):3148-3166.

17. Gogas BD, Farooq V, Serruys PW, Garcìa-Garcìa HM. Assessment of coronary atherosclerosis by IVUS and IVUS-based imaging modalities: progression and regression studies, tissue composition and beyond. The International Journal of Cardiovascular Imaging. 2011;27(2):225-237. Doi:10.1007/s10554-010-9791-0.

18. Pathan F, Negishi K. Prediction of cardiovascular outcomes by imaging coronary atherosclerosis. Cardiovascular Diagnosis and Therapy. 2016;6(4):322-339. Doi:10.21037/cdt.2015.12.08.

19. Ornish D, Scherwitz LW, Billings JH, et al. Intensive lifestyle changes for reversal of coronary heart disease: five-year follow-up of the Lifestyle Heart Trial. JAMA. 1998;280(23):2001–2007.

20. Qaseem A, Fihn SD, Dallas P, Williams S, Owens DK, Shekelle P. Management of stable ischemic heart disease: summary of a clinical practice guideline from the American College of Physicians/American College of Cardiology Foundation/American Heart Association/American Association for Thoracic Surgery/Preventive Cardiovascular Nurses

Association/Society of Thoracic Surgeons. Ann Intern Med. 2012;157(10):735–743.

21. Degrauwe S, Pilgrim T, Aminian A, Noble S, Meier P, Iglesias JF. Dual antiplatelet therapy for secondary prevention of coronary artery disease. Open Heart. 2017;4(2): e000651. doi:10.1136/openhrt-2017-000651.

22. Delui MH, Yari M, khouyinezhad G, Amini M, Bayazi MH. Comparison of Cardiac Rehabilitation Programs Combined with Relaxation and Meditation Techniques on Reduction of Depression and Anxiety of Cardiovascular Patients. The Open Cardiovascular Medicine Journal. 2013;7:99-103. doi:10.2174/1874192401307010099.

23. Raghuram N, Parachuri VR, Swarnagowri MV, et al. Yoga based cardiac rehabilitation after coronary artery bypass surgery: One-year results on LVEF, lipid profile and psychological states – A randomized controlled study. Indian Heart Journal. 2014;66(5):490-502. doi:10.1016/j.ihj.2014.08.007.

24. Gomes-Neto M, Rodrigues-Jr ES, Silva-Jr WM, Carvalho VO. Effects of Yoga in Patients with Chronic Heart Failure: A Meta-Analysis. Arquivos Brasileiros de Cardiologia. 2014;103(5):433-439. doi:10.5935/abc.20140149.

25. Lan C, Chen S-Y, Wong M-K, Lai JS. Tai Chi Chuan Exercise for Patients with Cardiovascular Disease. Evidence-based Complementary and Alternative Medicine□: eCAM. 2013;2013:983208. doi:10.1155/2013/983208.

26. Bruning RS, Sturek M. Benefits of exercise training on coronary blood flow in coronary artery disease patients. Progress in cardiovascular diseases. 2015;57(5):443-453. doi:10.1016/j.pcad.2014.10.006.

27. Yu C, Ji K, Cao H, et al. Effectiveness of acupuncture for angina pectoris: a systematic review of randomized controlled trials. BMC Complementary and Alternative Medicine. 2015;15:90. doi:10.1186/s12906-015-0586-7.

28. Tupule TH, Shah HM, Shah SJ, et al. Yogic exercises in the management of ischaemic heart disease. Indian Heart Journal. 1971;23(4):259–264.

29. Tupule TH, Shah HM, Shah SJ, et al. Yogic exercises in the management of ischaemic heart disease. Indian Heart Journal. 1971;23(4):259–264.

30. Hagins M, States R, Selfe T, et al. Effectiveness of Yoga for Hypertension: Systematic Review and Meta-Analysis Evidence-Based Complementary and Alternative Medicine. Volume 2013 (2013), Article ID 649836.

31. Wang J, Xiong X, Liu W (2013) Yoga for Essential Hypertension: A Systematic Review. PLoS ONE 8(10): e76357. https://doi.org/10.1371/journal.pone.0076357.

32. Okonta Nkechi. Does yoga therapy reduce blood pressure in patients with hypertension? An integrative review. Holist Nurs Pract 2012; 26: 137-141.

33. Tyagi A, Cohen M. Yoga and hypertension: a systematic review. Altern Ther Health Med. 2014 Mar-Apr;20(2):32-59.

34. Manchanda SC, Narang R, Reddy KS, Sachdeva U, Prabhakaran D, Dharmanand S, et al. Retardation of coronary atherosclerosis with yoga lifestyle intervention. J Assoc Physicians India. 2000;48:687–94.

35. Siu PM, Yu AP, Benzie IF, Woo J. Effects of 1-year yoga on cardiovascular risk factors in middle-aged and older adults with metabolic syndrome: a randomized trial. Diabetology & Metabolic Syndrome. 2015;7:40. doi:10.1186/s13098-015-0034-3.

36. Ross A., Friedmann E., Bevans M., Thomas S. National survey of yoga practitioners: mental and physical health benefits. Complementary Therapies in Medicine. 2013;21(4):313–323. doi: 10.1016/j.ctim.2013.04.001.

37. Ross A., Friedmann E., Bevans M., Thomas S. Frequency of yoga practice predicts health: results of a national survey of yoga practitioners. Evidence-based Complementary and Alternative Medicine. 2012;2012:10. doi: 10.1155/2012/983258.983258).

38. Olson K. L., Emery C. F. Mindfulness and weight loss: a systematic review. Psychosomatic Medicine. 2015;77(1):59–67.; Rioux JG, Ritenbaugh C. Narrative review of yoga intervention clinical trials including weight-related outcomes. Altern Ther Health Med. 2013 May-Jun;19(3):32-46.

39. Acharya BK, AK Upadhyay, Ruchita T Upadhyay,et al. Effect of Pranayama (voluntary regulated breathing) and Yogasana (yoga postures) on lipid profile in normal healthy junior footballers. Int J Yoga. 2010 Jul-Dec; 3(2): 70.

40. Yadav RK, Magan D, Yadav R, et al. High-density lipoprotein cholesterol increases following a short-term yoga-based lifestyle intervention: a non-pharmacological modulation. Acta Cardiol. 2014 Oct;69(5):543-9.

41. Gokal R, Shillito L, Maharaj SR. Positive impact of yoga and pranayam on obesity, hypertension, blood sugar, and cholesterol: a pilot assessment. J Altern Complement Med. 2007 Dec;13(10):1056-7.

42. Mahajan A., Reddy K., Sachdeva U. Lipid profile of coronary risk subjects following yogic lifestyle intervention. Indian Heart J. 1999;51:37–40.

43. Shantakumari N, Sequeira S, El deeb R. Effects of a yoga intervention on lipid profiles of diabetes patients with dyslipidemia. Indian Heart Journal. 2013;65(2):127-131. doi:10.1016/j.ihj.2013.02.010.

44. Innes KE, Selfe TK. Yoga for Adults with Type 2 Diabetes: A Systematic Review of Controlled Trials. Journal of Diabetes Research. 2016;2016:6979370. doi:10.1155/2016/6979370.

45. Kelly A McDermott, Mohan Raghavendra Rao, Raghuram Nagarathna, Elizabeth J Murphy, Adam Burke, Ramarao Hongasandra Nagendra and Frederick M Hecht. A yoga intervention for type 2 diabetes risk reduction: a pilot randomized controlled trial. BMC Complementary and Alternative Medicine. 201414:212.

46. Innes KE, Selfe TK. Yoga for Adults with Type 2 Diabetes: A Systematic Review of Controlled Trials. Journal of Diabetes Research. 2016;2016:6979370. doi:10.1155/2016/6979370.

47. Kerr D, Gillam E, Ryder J, Trowbridge S, et al. An Eastern art form for a Western disease: randomised controlled trial of yoga in patients with poorly controlled insulin-treated diabetes. Pract Diabetes Intern. 2002; 19:164–6.
48. Bock BC, Fava JL, Gaskins R, et al. Yoga as a complementary treatment for smoking cessation in women. J Womens Health (Larchmt) 2012;21(2):240–248.
49. L Carim Todd, S Mitchell, B Oken. Does yoga improve smoking cessation outcomes? A systematic review of the literature. BMC Complement Altern Med. 2012; 12(Suppl 1): P389. Published online 2012 Jun 12.
50. Shahab L, Sarkar BK, West R. The acute effects of yogic breathing exercises on craving and withdrawal symptoms in abstaining smokers. Psychopharmacology (Berl). 2013 Feb;225(4):875-82.
51. Klinsophon T, Thaveeratitham P, Sitthipornvorakul E, Janwantanakul P. Effect of exercise type on smoking cessation: a meta-analysis of randomized controlled trials. BMC Research Notes. 2017;10:442. doi:10.1186/s13104-017-2762-y.
52. Dick H. J. Thijssen,Andrew J. Maiorana, et al. Impact of inactivity and exercise on the vasculature in humans. Eur J Appl Physiol. 2010 Mar; 108(5): 845–875.
53. Chastin SFM, Palarea-Albaladejo J, et al. (2015) Combined Effects of Time Spent in Physical Activity, Sedentary Behaviors and Sleep on Obesity and Cardio-Metabolic Health Markers: A Novel Compositional Data Analysis Approach. PLoS ONE 10(10): e0139984.
54. Long R. Scientific keys volume I: the key muscles of hatha yoga. 3. Bandha: Yoga; 2006.
55. McCall T. Yoga as medicine: The yogic prescription for health and healing. 1. New York: Bantam Dell; 2007.
56. Ray US, Pathak A, Tomer OS. Hatha yoga practices: Energy expenditure, respiratory changes and intensity of exercise. Evid Based Complement Alternat Med. 2011; 2011:241294.
57. Sovová E, Čajka V, Pastucha D, et al. Positive effect of yoga on cardiorespiratory fitness: A pilot study. Int J Yoga. 2015 Jul-Dec;8(2):134-8.
58. Vijayaraghava A, Doreswamy V, Narasipur OS, Kunnavil R, Srinivasamurthy N. Effect of Yoga Practice on Levels of Inflammatory Markers After Moderate and Strenuous Exercise. Journal of Clinical and Diagnostic Research□: JCDR. 2015;9(6):CC08-CC12. doi:10.7860/JCDR/2015/12851.6021.
59. Kiecolt-Glaser JK, Christian L, Preston H, et al. Stress, Inflammation, and Yoga Practice. Psychosomatic medicine. 2010;72(2):113. doi:10.1097/PSY.0b013e3181cb9377.
60. Thirthalli J, Naveen GH, Rao MG, Varambally S, Christopher R, Gangadhar BN. Cortisol and antidepressant effects of yoga. Indian Journal of Psychiatry. 2013;55(Suppl 3):S405-S408. doi:10.4103/0019-5545.116315.

61. Yadav RK, Magan D, Mehta N, Sharma R, Mahapatra SC. Efficacy of a short-term yoga-based lifestyle intervention in reducing stress and inflammation: preliminary results. J Altern Complement Med. 2012 Jul;18(7):662-7. doi: 10.1089/acm.2011.0265.
62. Lau HL, Kwong JS, Yeung F, et al. Yoga for secondary prevention of coronary heart disease. Cochrane Database Syst Rev. 2012 Dec 12;12:CD009506.
63. Yadav A, Singh S, Singh KP. Role of Pranayama breathing exercises in rehabilitation of CAD patients - A pilot study. Indian J Tradit Knowledge. 2009;8:455–8.
64. Yadav A, Singh S, Singh K, Pai P. Effect of yoga regimen on lung functions including diffusion capacity in coronary artery disease patients: A randomized controlled study. International Journal of Yoga. 2015;8(1):62-67. doi:10.4103/0973-6131.146067.
65. Yogendra J, Yogendra H, Ambardekar S, et al. Beneficial effects of yoga lifestyle on reversibility of ischaemic heart disease: Caring Heart Project of International Board of Yoga. JAPI. 2004; 52:283.
66. Ramamurthy G, Trejo E, Faraone SV. Depression Treatment in Patients with Coronary Artery Disease: A Systematic Review. The Primary Care Companion for CNS Disorders. 2013;15(5):PCC.13r01509. doi:10.4088/PCC.13r01509.
67. Parswani MJ, Sharma MP, Iyengar S. Mindfulness-based stress reduction program in coronary heart disease: A randomized control trial. International Journal of Yoga. 2013;6(2):111-117. doi:10.4103/0973-6131.113405.
68. O'Connor GT, JE Buring, S Yusuf, et al. An overview of randomized trials of rehabilitation with exercise after myocardial infarction. Circulation 1989;80;234-244.
69. Raghuram N, Parachuri VR, Swarnagowri MV, et al. Yoga based cardiac rehabilitation after coronary artery bypass surgery: One-year results on LVEF, lipid profile and psychological states – A randomized controlled study. Indian Heart Journal. 2014;66(5):490-502. doi:10.1016/j.ihj.2014.08.007.

Congestive Heart Failure

Congestive heart failure (CHF) is a common cardiac disease[1]. It is estimated that it effects over 5.8 million people in the USA and over 23 million worldwide[2,3]. An American has a one in five risk of developing heart failure during his/her lifetime[4,5]. Heart failure is a deadly disease, with substantial morbidity and mortality. It is estimated that following a diagnosis, 30-day mortality is around 10%, 1-year mortality is 20–30%, and 5-year mortality is 45–60%[5]. As the heart failure gets severe, life expectancy of CHF patients becomes comparable to those with aggressive cancers[6]. Patients with heart failure have multiple symptoms, including fatigue, dyspnea, fluid retention, and cachexia. Despite symptomatic treatment to relieve symptoms and the use of several classes of drugs to improve the prognosis, including implantable devices[7,8], heart failure continues to be responsible for almost 1 million hospitalizations annually and accounting for over 6.5 million hospital days[9]. Worldwide, the prevalence of heart failure has continued to increase, and has become a major global health problem[10]. Complementary and alternative medicine has been used by patients with heart failure[11,12]. The role of yoga in the management of heart failure has also been investigated in several trials[13].

Yoga and Congestive Heart Failure

When yoga was combined with standard care, an 8-week regimen of yoga in patients with CHF resulted in significant improvements. The study involved 19 patients with Grade I-III heart failure (with a mean ejection fraction of 25%). Nine patients were randomized to yoga and ten to standard medical care. At the end of the study, patients in the yoga group showed significantly improved graded exercise time and peak vo2. The yoga group patients also had significant reductions in serum levels of IL-6 and hsCRP and an increase in extracellular superoxide dismutase. Minnesota Living with Heart Failure Questionnaire scores improved by 25.7% in the yoga group and by only 2.9% in the medical treatment group[14].

In a study of 15 stable heart failure patients, given 8 weeks of yoga classes, the researchers reported a significant improvement in endurance and strength. Balance and overall mood/wellbeing improved. Symptom stability, a subscale of quality of life, improved significantly. No adverse effects were noted[15].

Pullen and group recruited 38 African Americans (plus one Asian and one Caucasian) with heart failure and randomly assigned them to a yoga group (21 patients) and a control group (19 patients). Both groups also followed a home walk program. At the end of the study, the yoga group showed improvements in flexibility, treadmill time, peak vo2, and IL-6, CRP, EC-SOD biomarkers. Quality of life was also improved in the yoga group[16].

A meta-analysis of two major studies revealed a 22% improvement in peak vo2 during cardiopulmonary exercise testing in the yoga group, indicating an increased exercise capacity. There was also a major improvement noted in the quality of life by 24% using the Minnesota Living with Heart Failure Questionnaire[17].

In a recent study of 130 (NYHA I-II) heart failure patients, randomization was done either to the 12-week yoga plus standard therapy (65 patients) or standard therapy (65 patients). In the yoga group, 44 patients and in the control group, 48 patients completed the study. The yoga group were noted to have a significant decrease in heart rate, blood pressure and rate pressure product compared to control group. Also, LFnu and LF-HF ratio decreased significantly and HFnu increased significantly in yoga group compared to control group. (spectral heart rate variability measures low-frequency (LF)nu and high-frequency (HF)nu) These changes are consistent with an improvement in the parasympathetic activity and a decrease in the sympathetic activity in the yoga group patients[18].

Conclusion

Congestive heart failure patients do better with yoga practice.

References

1. Bui AL, Horwich TB, Fonarow GC. Epidemiology and risk profile of heart failure. Nature reviews Cardiology. 2011;8(1):30-41. doi:10.1038/nrcardio.2010.165.

2. Lloyd-Jones D, et al. Heart disease and stroke statistics—2010 update: a report from the American Heart Association. Circulation. 2010;121:e46–e215.
3. McMurray JJ, Petrie MC, Murdoch DR, Davie AP. Clinical epidemiology of heart failure: public and private health burden. Eur Heart J. 1998;19 (Suppl P):P9–P16.
4. Lloyd-Jones D, et al. Heart disease and stroke statistics—2010 update: a report from the American Heart Association. Circulation. 2010;121:e46–e215.
5. Levy D, et al. Long-term trends in the incidence of and survival with heart failure. N Engl J Med. 2002;347:1397–1402.
6. Stewart S, MacIntyre K, Hole DJ, Capewell S, McMurray JJ. More 'malignant' than cancer? Five-year survival following a first admission for heart failure. Eur J Heart Fail. 2001;3:315–322.
7. Dunlay SM, Pereira NL, Kushwaha SS. Contemporary Strategies in the Diagnosis and Management of Heart Failure. Mayo Clinic proceedings. 2014;89(5):662-676. doi:10.1016/j.mayocp.2014.01.004.
8. Bernardo BC, Blaxall BC. From Bench to Bedside: New approaches to therapeutic discovery for heart failure. Heart, lung & circulation. 2016;25(5):425-434. doi:10.1016/j.hlc.2016.01.002.
9. Gheorghiade M, Vaduganathan M, Fonarow GC, Bonow RO. Rehospitalization for heart failure: problems and perspectives. J Am Coll Cardiol. 2013 Jan 29;61(4):391-403. doi: 10.1016/j.jacc.2012.09.038. Epub 2012 Dec 5.
10. Norton C, Georgiopoulou VV, Kalogeropoulos AP, Butler J. Epidemiology and cost of advanced heart failure. Prog Cardiovasc Dis. 2011 Sep-Oct;54(2):78-85. doi: 10.1016/j.pcad.2011.04.002.
11. Albert N, Rathman L, Ross D, Walker D, Bena J, McIntyre S, Philip D, Siedlecki S, Lovelace R, Fogarty A. et al. Predictors of Over-the-Counter Drug and Herbal Therapies Use in Elderly Patients with Heart Failure. J Card Fail. 2009;15(7):600–606. doi: 10.1016/j.cardfail.2009.02.001.
12. Pan L, Yan J, Guo Y, Yan J. Effects of Tai Chi training on exercise capacity and quality of life in patients with chronic heart failure: a meta-analysis. Eur J Heart Fail. 2013 Mar;15(3):316-23. doi: 10.1093/eurjhf/hfs170. Epub 2012 Oct 25.
13. Kubo A, Hung YY, Ritterman J. Yoga for heart failure patients: a feasibility pilot study with a multiethnic population. Int J Yoga Therap. 2011;(21):77-83.
14. Pullen PR, Nagamia SH, Mehta PK, Thompson WR, Benardot D, Hammoud R, Parrott JM, Sola S, Khan BV. Effects of yoga on inflammation and exercise capacity in patients with chronic heart failure. J Card Fail. 2008 Jun;14(5):407-13.
15. Howie-Esquivel J, et al. Yoga in heart failure patients: a pilot study. J Card Fail. 2010.
16. Pullen PR, Thompson WR, Benardot D, Brandon LJ, Mehta PK, Rifai L, Vadnais DS, Parrott JM, Khan BV. Benefits of yoga for African

American heart failure patients. Med Sci Sports Exerc. 2010 Apr;42(4):651-7. doi: 10.1249/MSS.0b013e3181bf24c4.

17. Gomes-Neto M, Rodrigues-Jr ES, Silva-Jr WM, Carvalho VO. Effects of Yoga in Patients with Chronic Heart Failure: A Meta-Analysis. Arquivos Brasileiros de Cardiologia. 2014;103(5):433-439. doi:10.5935/abc.20140149.

18. Krishna BH, et al. Effect of yoga therapy on heart rate, blood pressure and cardiac autonomic function in heart failure. J Clin Diagn Res. 2014 Jan;8(1):14-6. doi: 10.7860/JCDR/2014/7844.3983. Epub 2014 Jan 12.

Depression

Major depression is a common mental disorder[1]. It is characterized by a depressed mood and/or loss of interest or pleasure in life activities for at least 2 weeks. Symptoms may include depressed mood most of the day, diminished interest or pleasure in all or most activities, significant unintentional weight loss or gain, insomnia or sleeping too much, agitation or psychomotor retardation (noticed by others), fatigue or loss of energy, feelings of worthlessness or excessive guilt., diminished ability to think or concentrate, or indecisiveness, and recurrent thoughts of death[2]. Major depression has a high rate of co-morbidity with other conditions, greatly impairing the daily functioning and quality of life of these patients[3]. It is often associated with alcohol, drug and smoking addictions, and sexual dysfunction[4]. It is estimated that 6.7% of all American adults (16.2 million) aged 18 or older had at least one major depressive episode in 2015[5]. It is more common in those who are unmarried, separated, or divorced and those without intact families[6]. Worldwide, almost 300 million people are affected[7].

Antidepressant therapy remains associated with an unacceptable rate of non-efficacy, drug resistance[8], polypharmacy[9] non-compliance, relapses and medication cost increases[10]. Complementary treatment modalities have shown benefit for several mental and associated physical health symptoms, functioning, self-care, and overall quality of life[11]. Yoga, a complementary practice, has also been investigated in several psychiatric conditions[12] including in the adjunctive management of depression, with good therapeutic results[13,14].

Yoga and Depression

Depression has attracted major scientific scrutiny by medical researchers[15]. In most studies, yoga therapy has been successful in positively modulating the various facets of depression[16-19].

In a study of young adults with self-reported depression, a significant reduction in depression scores was noted[20]. In this study, 28 volunteers ages 18 to 29 with mild depression were recruited. The yoga group, attended two 1-hour Iyengar yoga classes each week for 5 consecutive weeks. Their outcomes were measured using Beck Depression Inventory, State-Trait Anxiety Inventory, Profile of Mood States, and morning cortisol levels. The yoga recruits reported decrease in symptoms of depression and trait anxiety. They also experienced decreased levels of negative mood and fatigue following the yoga classes.

Yogic breathing improved emotions and reduced sadness in young adults with depression[21]. Yoga therapy has also been shown to alleviate depression in older individuals[22]. In women with major depression, increased connectedness and decreased rumination was noted with yoga therapy[23]. Its benefit has also been noted in pregnant women prone to [24] as well as in those suffering from prenatal[25] and postpartum depression[26].

Yoga therapy has been salutary in depression associated with a wide variety of physical and mental conditions[27-32]. These include depression associated with breast cancer[33], low back pain[34], post stroke hemiparesis[35], multiple sclerosis[36], Parkinson's disease[37], atrial fibrillation[38], heart failure[39], hospice care[40], and chronic obstructive pulmonary disease[41]. Yoga has reduced depression in patients with associated mental co-morbidities, especially anxiety[42], and post-traumatic stress disorder[43]. Yoga therapy improves several psychological parameters including depression in inpatients in a rehabilitation and complex continuing care hospital[44]. Yoga along with psycho-education has resulted in more remissions in depressed patients with long term symptoms[45]. A recent study has confirmed sustained beneficial effects of yoga in a depressed female population[46] Yoga also appears to reduce depression in caregivers[47,48]. Mindfulness meditation may help prevent depression relapses[49].

Depression has an association with increased cortisol levels[50] and low brain derived neurotrophic factor[51]. These are improved by yoga practice[52]. Yoga may also be enhancing positive neuroplasticity, as evidenced by an increase in hippocampal volume[53] and improved cognition[54]. There is a decrease in the sympathetic tone and a shift of the autonomic balance to the parasympathetic side[55]. Many other bio-neuro-chemical changes also play a role in the yoga associated benefit in depression[56-58].

Studies have shown that yoga is feasible and acceptable in patients with depression[59].

Conclusion

Yoga is a good complimentary treatment for depression.

References

1. Kessler RC, Bromet EJ. The epidemiology of depression across cultures. Annual review of public health. 2013;34:119-138. doi:10.1146/annurev-publhealth-031912-114409.
2. samhsa.gov – accessed 9/1/17.
3. Kessler RC1, Berglund P, Demler O et al. The epidemiology of major depressive disorder: results from the National Comorbidity Survey Replication (NCS-R). JAMA. 2003 Jun 18;289(23):3095-105.
4. Sihvola E, Rose RJ, Dick DM, Pulkkinen L, Marttunen M, Kaprio J. Early-onset depressive disorders predict the use of addictive substances in adolescence: a prospective study of adolescent Finnish twins. Addiction. 2008 Dec;103(12):2045-53. doi: 10.1111/j.1360-0443.2008.02363.x. Epub 2008 Oct 8.
5. nimh.nih.gov/health/statistics/major-depression.shtml – accessed 1/21/18.
6. Evelyn BrometEmail author, Laura Helena Andrade, Irving Hwang et al. Cross-national epidemiology of DSM-IV major depressive episode. BMC Medicine20119:90.
7. who.int/mediacentre/factsheets/fs369/en/ - accessed 1/21/18.
8. Al-Harbi KS. Treatment-resistant depression: therapeutic trends, challenges, and future directions. Patient preference and adherence. 2012;6:369-388. doi:10.2147/PPA.S29716.
9. Covadonga M., Díaz-Caneja, Ana Espliego, Mara Parellada, Celso Arango, Carmen Moreno. Polypharmacy with antidepressants in children and adolescents. International Journal of Neuropsychopharmacology, Volume 17, Issue 7, 1 July 2014, Pages 1063–1082.
10. Keller MB. McCullough JP. Klein DN, et al. A comparison of nefazodone, the cognitive behavioral–analysis system of psychotherapy, and their combination for the treatment of chronic depression. N Engl J Med. 2000;342(20):1462–1470.
11. Qureshi NA, Al-Bedah AM. Mood disorders and complementary and alternative medicine: a literature review. Neuropsychiatric Disease and Treatment. 2013;9:639-658. doi:10.2147/NDT.S43419.
12. Klatte R, Pabst S, Beelmann A, Rosendahl J. The Efficacy of Body-Oriented Yoga in Mental Disorders: A Systematic Review and Meta-Analysis. Deutsches Ärzteblatt International. 2016;113(12):195-202. doi:10.3238/arztebl.2016.0195.;Cramer et al, 2017.
13. Chu IH, Wu WL, Lin IM, Chang YK, Lin YJ, Yang PC. Effects of Yoga on Heart Rate Variability and Depressive Symptoms in Women: A

Randomized Controlled Trial. J Altern Complement Med. 2017 Apr;23(4):310-316. doi: 10.1089/acm.2016.0135. Epub 2017 Jan 4.

14. Bonura KB1, Tenenbaum G. Effects of yoga on psychological health in older adults. J Phys Act Health. 2014 Sep;11(7):1334-41. doi: 10.1123/jpah.2012-0365. Epub 2013 Dec 20.

15. Cramer H, Lauche R, Dobos G. Characteristics of randomized controlled trials of yoga: a bibliometric analysis. BMC Complementary and Alternative Medicine. 2014;14:328. doi:10.1186/1472-6882-14-328.

16. Pilkington K, Kirkwood G, Rampes H, et al. Yoga for depression: The research evidence. J Affect Disord. 2005;89:13–24.

17. Kinser PA, Goehler L, Taylor AG. How Might Yoga Help Depression? A Neurobiological Perspective. Explore (New York, NY). 2012;8(2):118-126.

18. Uebelacker LA, Epstein-Lubow G, Gaudiano BA, et al. Hatha yoga for depression: critical review of the evidence for efficacy, plausible mechanisms of action, and directions for future research. J Psychiatr Pract. 2010 Jan;16(1):22-33.

19. Uebelacker LA, Broughton MK. Yoga for Depression and Anxiety: A Review of Published Research and Implications for Healthcare Providers. R I Med J (2013). 2016 Mar 1;99(3):20-2.

20. Woolery A, Myers H, Sternlieb B, et al. A yoga intervention for young adults with elevated symptoms of depression. Altern Ther Health Med. 2004 Mar-Apr;10(2):60-3.

21. Falsafi N. A Randomized Controlled Trial of Mindfulness Versus Yoga: Effects on Depression and/or Anxiety in College Students. J Am Psychiatr Nurses Assoc. 2016 Nov;22(6):483-497.

22. Bonura KB, Tenenbaum G. Effects of yoga on psychological health in older adults. J Phys Act Health. 2014 Sep;11(7):1334-41.

23. Kinser PA, Bourguignon C, Taylor AG, et al. "A Feeling of Connectedness": Perspectives on a Gentle Yoga Intervention for Women with Major Depression. Issues in mental health nursing. 2013;34(6):402-411.

24. (Muzik M, Hamilton SE, Rosenblum KL, et al. Mindfulness yoga during pregnancy for psychiatrically at-risk women: Preliminary results from a pilot feasibility study. Complement Ther Clin Pract. 2012;18(4):235–40.

25. Babbar S, Shyken J. Yoga in Pregnancy. Clin Obstet Gynecol. 2016 Sep;59(3):600-12.

26. Buttner MM, Brock RL, O'Hara MW, et al. Efficacy of yoga for depressed postpartum women: A randomized controlled trial. Complement Ther Clin Pract. 2015 May;21(2):94-100.

27. Sharma VK, Das S, Mondal S, et al. Effect of Sahaj Yoga on neuro-cognitive functions in patients suffering from major depression. Indian J Physiol Pharmacol. 2006 Oct-Dec;50(4):375-83.

28. Desveaux L, Lee A, Goldstein R, Brooks D. Yoga in the Management of Chronic Disease: A Systematic Review and Meta-analysis. Med Care. 2015 Jul;53(7):653-61.

29. Telles S, Pathak S, Kumar A, et al. Influence of Intensity and Duration of Yoga on Anxiety and Depression Scores Associated with Chronic Illness. Ann Med Health Sci Res. 2015 Jul-Aug;5(4):260-5.
30. Gong H, Ni C, Shen X, et al. Yoga for prenatal depression: a systematic review and meta-analysis. BMC Psychiatry. 2015 Feb 5;15:14.
31. Rogers KA, MacDonald M. Therapeutic Yoga: Symptom Management for Multiple Sclerosis. J Altern Complement Med. 2015 Nov;21(11):655-9.
32. Brinzo JA, Crenshaw JT, Thomas L, et al. The effect of yoga on depression and pain in adult patients with chronic low back pain: a systematic review protocol. JBI Database System Rev Implement Rep. 2016 Jan;14(1):56-66.
33. Rao RM, Nagendra HR, Raghuram N, et al. Influence of yoga on mood states, distress, quality of life and immune outcomes in early stage breast cancer patients undergoing surgery. Int J Yoga. 2008 Jan;1(1):11-20.
34. Tekur P, Nagarathna R, Chametcha S, et al. A comprehensive yoga programs improves pain, anxiety and depression in chronic low back pain patients more than exercise: an RCT. Complement Ther Med. 2012 Jun;20(3):107-18.
35. Chan W, Immink MA, Hillier S. Yoga and exercise for symptoms of depression and anxiety in people with poststroke disability: a randomized, controlled pilot trial. Altern Ther Health Med. 2012 May-Jun;18(3):34-43.
36. Chobe S, Bhargav H, Raghuram N, et al. Effect of integrated Yoga and Physical therapy on audiovisual reaction time, anxiety and depression in patients with chronic multiple sclerosis: a pilot study. J Complement Integr Med. 2016 Sep 1;13(3):301-309.
37. Sharma N., Robbins K., Wagner K., et al. A randomized controlled pilot study of the therapeutic effects of yoga in people with Parkinson's disease. International Journal of Yoga. 2015;8(1):74–79.
38. Lakkireddy D, Donita Atkins, Jayasree Pillarisetti, et al. Effect of Yoga on Arrhythmia Burden, Anxiety, Depression, and Quality of Life in Paroxysmal Atrial Fibrillation. The YOGA My Heart Study. J Am Coll Cardiol. 2013; 61(11):1177-1182.
39. Hägglund E, Hagerman I, Dencker K, Strömberg A. Effects of yoga versus hydrotherapy training on health-related quality of life and exercise capacity in patients with heart failure: A randomized controlled study. Eur J Cardiovasc Nurs. 2017 Jan 1:1474515117690297.
40. Ramanathan M, Bhavanani AB, Trakroo M. Effect of a 12-week yoga therapy program on mental health status in elderly women inmates of a hospice. Int J Yoga. 2017 Jan-Apr;10(1):24-28.
41. Ranjita R, Badhai S, Hankey A, et al. A randomized controlled study on assessment of health status, depression, and anxiety in coal miners with chronic obstructive pulmonary disease following yoga training. International Journal of Yoga. 2016;9(2):137-144.

42. Tolbaños Roche L, Miró Barrachina MT, Ibáñez Fernández I. Effect of 'Exercise Without Movement' yoga method on mindfulness, anxiety and depression. Complement Ther Clin Pract. 2016 Nov;25:136-141.
43. Hilton L, Maher AR, Colaiaco B, et al. Meditation for Posttraumatic Stress: Systematic Review and Meta-analysis. Psychol Trauma. 2016 Aug 18.
44. Curtis K, Kuluski K, Bechsgaard G, et al. Evaluation of a Specialized Yoga Program for Persons Admitted to a Complex Continuing Care Hospital: A Pilot Study. Evid Based Complement Alternat Med. 2016;2016:6267879.
45. Butler LD, Waelde LC, Hastings TA, et al. Meditation with yoga, group therapy with hypnosis, and psychoeducation for long-term depressed mood: a randomized pilot trial. J Clin Psychol. 2008 Jul;64(7):806-20.
46. Kinser PA, Elswick RK, Kornstein S. Potential long-term effects of a mind-body intervention for women with major depressive disorder: Sustained mental health improvements with a pilot yoga intervention. Archives of psychiatric nursing. 2014;28(6):377-383.
47. Lavretsky H, Siddarth P, Nazarian N, et al. A pilot study of yogic meditation for family dementia caregivers with depressive symptoms: Effects on mental health, cognition, and telomerase activity. International journal of geriatric psychiatry. 2013;28(1):57-65.
48. Umadevi P, Ramachandra S, Varambally S, et al. Effect of yoga therapy on anxiety and depressive symptoms and quality-of-life among caregivers of in-patients with neurological disorders at a tertiary care center in India: A randomized controlled trial. Indian J Psychiatry [serial online] 2013 [cited 2017 Feb 5];55, Suppl S3:385-9.
49. Edenfield TM, Saeed SA. An update on mindfulness meditation as a self-help treatment for anxiety and depression. Psychology Research and Behavior Management. 2012;5:131-141. doi:10.2147/PRBM.S34937.
50. Stetler C, Miller GE. Depression and Hypothalamic-Pituitary-Adrenal Activation: A Quantitative Summary of Four Decades of Research. Psychosom Med. 2011;73(2):114–26.
51. Naveen GH, Varambally S, Thirthalli J, et al. Serum cortisol and BDNF in patients with major depression-effect of yoga. Int Rev Psychiatry. 2016 Jun;28(3):273-8.
52. Naveen GH, Varambally S, Thirthalli J, et al. Serum cortisol and BDNF in patients with major depression-effect of yoga. Int Rev Psychiatry. 2016 Jun;28(3):273-8.
53. Hariprasad VR, Varambally S, Shivakumar V, et al. Yoga increases the volume of the hippocampus in elderly subjects. Indian J Psychiatry. 2013;55 (Suppl 3):S394–6.
54. Sharma VK, Das S, Mondal S, et al. Effect of Sahaj Yoga on neuro-cognitive functions in patients suffering from major depression. Indian J Physiol Pharmacol. 2006 Oct-Dec;50(4):375-83.
55. Bharshankar JR, Mandape AD, Phatak MS, et al. Autonomic Functions In Raja-yoga Meditators. Indian J Physiol Pharmacol. 2015 Oct-Dec;59(4):396-401.

56. Streeter C. C., Jensen J. E., Perlmutter R. M. Yoga asana sessions increase brain GABA levels: a pilot study. J. Altern. Complement. Med. 2007;13, 419–42610.1089/acm.2007.6338.

57. Yoshihara K, Hiramoto T, Sudo N, et al. Profile of mood states and stress-related biochemical indices in long-term yoga practitioners. Biopsychosoc Med. 2011 Jun 3;5(1):6.

58. Jayaram N, Varambally S, Behere RV, et al. Effect of yoga therapy on plasma oxytocin and facial emotion recognition deficits in patients of schizophrenia. Indian J Psychiatry. 2013;55(Suppl 3):S409–13.

59. Kinser PA, Bourguignon C, Whaley D, Hauenstein E, Taylor AG. Feasibility, acceptability, and effects of gentle Hatha yoga for women with major depression: Findings from a randomized controlled mixed-methods study. Archives of psychiatric nursing. 2013;27(3):137-147. doi:10.1016/j.apnu.2013.01.003.

Diabetes Mellitus

Diabetes mellitus is a common disease. In the US, in 2015, there were 30.3 million Americans who had diabetes. This number accounted for 9.4% of the population. Of this population, 23.1 million were diagnosed while 7.2 million remained undiagnosed[1]. Prediabetes affects another 84.1 million Americans, who are 18 or above in age. In 2015, diabetes was the 7th leading cause of death in the US. It is estimated that about 1.5 million Americans are diagnosed with diabetes every year. The prevalence of diabetes is increasing, and it is estimated that 21% of the US population will be diabetic by the year 2050[2].

Of those with diabetes, 95% have type II diabetes, with only 5% having type I diabetes[3]. Type 2 diabetic patients typically have combinations of decreased insulin secretion and decreased insulin sensitivity (insulin resistance), while those with type 1 show destruction of pancreatic β-cells[4]. Cardiovascular disease is the most common cause of death in these patients[5]. Diabetics also suffer from neuropathy, blindness, kidney failure, and lower limb amputations[6-8]. Worldwide, there were 422 million diabetics in 2012, and these numbers are on the increase[9]. Almost 1.6 million deaths around the world were attributed to diabetes in 2015.

According to the American Diabetic Association, an A1c value of ≥6.5% or fasting glucose ≥126 mg/dL or 2-h glucose ≥200 mg/dL is consistent with a diagnosis of diabetes mellitus. Patients with an A1c in the range of 5.7% to 6.4% or a fasting glucose of 100 to 125 mg/dL or 2-h glucose of 140 to 199 mg/dL, are at an increased risk for diabetes mellitus and are classified as suffering from prediabetes[10].

Patients with diabetes mellitus may be asymptomatic, and remain undiagnosed for many years. Suggestive symptoms include, polyuria, polydipsia, polyphagia, weight loss, blurred vision, lower extremity paresthesias, or recurrent yeast infections[11]. Treatment should be carried out as per the recommendations of the American Diabetic Association -

Standards of Medical Care in Diabetes[12]. Yogic practices are also beneficial in patients with diabetes mellitus.

Yoga and Diabetes Mellitus

In a review of 70 studies of yoga practice in diabetics, researchers found beneficial changes in glucose tolerance and insulin sensitivity, lipid profiles, blood pressure and anthropometric characteristics. Several other risk factors for cardiovascular diseases were also improved, including oxidative stress, coagulation profiles, sympathetic activation, cardiovagal function, and numerous clinical endpoints[13].

In another review of several trials involving 2170 participants, researchers concluded that yoga modalities improved glycemic control and decreased insulin resistance, improved lipid levels (reductions in levels of total cholesterol, low-density lipoprotein cholesterol, very low-density lipoprotein cholesterol, and triglycerides, and increases in high-density lipoprotein cholesterol), reduced blood pressure and improved measures of body composition. (reductions in weight, body mass index and waist-hip ratio)[14]. Yoga interventions varied from study to study, but on an average, included 1-2 sessions per week for 12 weeks, and daily home practice. Most studies incorporated active yoga poses, in addition to breathing exercises and meditation/relaxation.

In a more recent review, of 12 randomized controlled trials with a total of 864 patients, yoga practice significantly decreased fasting blood glucose, post-prandial blood glucose, HbA1c, triglycerides and low density lipoprotein cholesterol levels, and increased high density lipoprotein cholesterol levels in patients with type 2 diabetes mellitus[15].

Yoga also helps in weight control and obesity and diabetes are intricately linked[16]. The beneficial effects of yoga in weight control are discussed in a subsequent chapter. In addition to improving diabetes and reducing the risk factors for cardiovascular disease, yoga also has a beneficial effect of several other complications of diabetes mellitus. Neuropathic pain in these patients show an improvement, with reduction in symptoms after 30–40 minutes of yoga, daily for 40 days[17].

Adding yoga to the usual treatment of diabetes also results in an improvement in the quality of life of these patients[18].

Conclusion

Yoga practice is helpful for patients with diabetes mellitus.

References

1. http://www.diabetes.org/diabetes-basics/statistics/?referrer=https://www.google.com/- accessed 1/1/18.
2. Boyle JP, Thompson TJ, Gregg EW, Barker LE, Williamson DF. Projection of the year 2050 burden of diabetes in the US adult population: dynamic modeling of incidence, mortality, and prediabetes prevalence. Popul Health Metr 2010;8:29.
3. (http://www.diabetes.org/diabetes-basics/statistics/infographics.html?referrer=https://www.google.com/)
4. The Committee of the Japan Diabetes Society on the Diagnostic Criteria of Diabetes Mellitus, Seino Y, Nanjo K, et al. Report of the Committee on the Classification and Diagnostic Criteria of Diabetes Mellitus. Journal of Diabetes Investigation. 2010;1(5):212-228. doi:10.1111/j.2040-1124.2010.00074.x.
5. Go AS, Mozaffarian D, Roger VL, et al. .; American Heart Association Statistics Committee and Stroke Statistics Subcommittee . Executive summary: heart disease and stroke statistics--2013 update: a report from the American Heart Association. Circulation 2013;127:143–152.
6. Sarwar N, Gao P, Seshasai SR, Gobin R, Kaptoge S, Di Angelantonio et al. Diabetes mellitus, fasting blood glucose concentration, and risk of vascular disease: a collaborative meta-analysis of 102 prospective studies. Emerging Risk Factors Collaboration. Lancet. 2010; 26;375:2215-2222.
7. Bourne RR, Stevens GA, White RA, Smith JL, Flaxman SR, Price H et al. Causes of vision loss worldwide, 1990-2010: a systematic analysis. Lancet Global Health 2013;1:e339-e349.
8. 2014 USRDS annual data report: Epidemiology of kidney disease in the United States. United States Renal Data System. National Institutes of Health, National Institute of Diabetes and Digestive and Kidney Diseases, Bethesda, MD, 2014:188–210.
9. http://www.who.int/mediacentre/factsheets/fs312/en/ - accessed 1/1/18.
10. American Diabetes Association Standards of medical care in diabetes—2015. Diabetes Care 2015;38(Suppl. 1):S1–S89.
11. https://emedicine.medscape.com/article/117853-clinical - accessed 1/2/18.

12. https://professional.diabetes.org/content-page/standards-medical-care-diabetes. – accessed 1/3/18.
13. Innes KE, Bourguignon C, Taylor AG. Risk indices associated with the insulin resistance syndrome, cardiovascular disease and possible protection with yoga: a systematic review. J Am Board Fam Pract. 2005;18:491–519. doi: 10.3122/jabfm.18.6.491.
14. Innes KE, Selfe TK. Yoga for Adults with Type 2 Diabetes: A Systematic Review of Controlled Trials. Journal of Diabetes Research. 2016;2016:6979370. doi:10.1155/2016/6979370.
15. Cui J, Yan J, Yan L, Pan L, Le J, Guo Y. Effects of yoga in adults with type 2 diabetes mellitus: A meta-analysis. Journal of Diabetes Investigation. 2017;8(2):201-209. doi:10.1111/jdi.12548.
16. Eckel RH, Kahn SE, Ferrannini E, et al. Obesity and Type 2 Diabetes: What Can Be Unified and What Needs to Be Individualized? The Journal of Clinical Endocrinology and Metabolism. 2011;96(6):1654-1663. doi:10.1210/jc.2011-0585.
17. Malhotra V., Singh S., Tandon O.P., Madhu S.V., Prasad A., Sharma S.B. (2002) Effect of Yoga asanas on nerve conduction in type 2 diabetes. Indian J Physiol Pharmacol 46: 298–306.
18. Keerthi GS, Pal P, Pal GK, Sahoo JP, Sridhar MG, Balachander J. Effect of 12 Weeks of Yoga Therapy on Quality of Life and Indian Diabetes Risk Score in Normotensive Indian Young Adult Prediabetics and Diabetics: Randomized Control Trial. Journal of Clinical and Diagnostic Research: JCDR. 2017;11(9):CC10-CC14. doi:10.7860/JCDR/2017/29307.10633.

Drug Addiction

The American Society of Addiction defines addiction as "a primary, chronic disease of brain reward, motivation, memory and related circuitry. Dysfunction in these circuits leads to characteristic biological, psychological, social and spiritual manifestations. This is reflected in an individual pathologically pursuing reward and/or relief by substance use and other behaviors. Addiction is characterized by inability to consistently abstain, impairment in behavioral control, craving, diminished recognition of significant problems with one's behaviors and interpersonal relationships, and a dysfunctional emotional response. Like other chronic diseases, addiction often involves cycles of relapse and remission. Without treatment or engagement in recovery activities, addiction is progressive and can result in disability or premature death"[1]. The World Health Organization estimates that the global burden of disease attributable to addiction amounts to 5.4% of the total[2]. Common addictions include those to nicotine, recreational substances such as marijuana, heroin, prescription drugs and alcohol. Prescription pain killers and opioids (includes heroin and prescription drugs such as oxycodone, hydrocodone, codeine, morphine, fentanyl and others) abuse or addiction was recorded in 20.5 million Americans 12 or older, in 2015[3]. Drug overdose is the leading cause of accidental death in the US. In 2015, there were 52,404 lethal drug overdoses. Prescription pain relievers were responsible for 20,101 overdose deaths and heroin for 12,990 overdose deaths[4].

Several medications are available to treat tobacco use disorders (nicotine replacement, bupropion, and varenicline), alcohol use disorders (naltrexone and acamprosate), and opioid use disorders (methadone and buprenorphine)[5,6]. Treatment also usually includes behavioral therapy (such as cognitive-behavioral therapy or contingency management)[7]. However, relapse rates remain as high as 80-95% in the first year after alcohol or tobacco cessation[8]. Complementary modalities have also been tried[9]. Yoga is also being used[10].

Yoga and Addiction

The benefits of yoga in alcohol abuse and smoking addiction is discussed under their own heading in this book. However, a few studies on these topics are presented here.

Smoking:

In an 8-week study, fifty-five women (post group-based cognitive behavioral therapy for smoking cessation), were randomized to a twice-weekly program of Vinyasa yoga or a control group attending a general health and wellness program. At the end of the treatment, researchers found that yoga practitioners had a higher abstinence rate than controls, and this rate remained higher at six months. The yoga group also showed reduced anxiety and improvements in perceived health and well-being when compared to controls[11]. In a review of four studies, Todd and associates found that the practice of yoga helped smokers quit. The yoga practitioners had increased desire and motivation to quit smoking. They had fewer urges to smoke and reduced temptations to smoke[12]. Mindfulness training has also been effective for smoking cessation[13].

Alcohol:

Hallgren and group randomized 18 alcohol dependent individuals into weekly group yoga for 10 weeks or treatment as usual groups. At the end of the study, the yoga group reduced alcohol consumption to a greater extent, when compared to the control group[14].

In women, age 18 to 65 years, suffering from PTSD, yoga intervention consisting of 12 Kripalu-based Hatha yoga sessions of 75 minutes each, resulted in a trend toward decreased alcohol use, when compared to the control group[15].

Drugs

An early study showed that hath yoga may help patients with drug addiction as much as traditional psychodynamic group therapy[16].

Zhuang and group[17] randomized seventy-five women aged 20-37 years undergoing inpatient detoxification for heroin dependence, into an intervention or a control group. The interventions group was given a 6-month yoga intervention in addition to hospital routine care, while the control group received hospital routine care only. They (most used injectable heroin) all suffered from poor mood and poor quality of life. The investigators found that yoga group, with yoga therapy, showed a significant improvement in mood status and quality of life over time compared to the control group.

In another study, Devi and associates[18] randomized a group of patients with substance use disorder into a yoga group (daily yoga sessions for 4 weeks) and a control group. Depressive symptoms improved significantly in the yoga group over the 4 weeks. There was an improvement in the quality of life domains of physical, psychological and social health, in the intervention group.

Sudarshan Kriya Yoga was studied with a treatment-as-usual control group. The eighty-four participants were already receiving buprenorphine for treatment of opiate dependence. Assessments were made at 3 and 6 months follow-up. The yoga group, compared to treatment-as-usual group, had better outcomes in the physical, psychological and environmental quality of life[19].

Yogic practice has helped patients with substance abuse in a pilot program that studied the effect of Kundalini based residential yoga treatment. The participants were a group of eight patients with a variety of substance use disorders (alcohol, opiates and barbiturates). They practiced Kundalini yoga for a period of 90 days. Compared to baseline values, the intervention group showed improvement in self-reported symptoms and problem severity, as well as the quality of recovery, though perceived stress did not change over the course of yoga intervention[20].

An efficacy trial on 168 adults with substance use disorders found that mindfulness based relapse prevention (MBRP) intervention group, compared to a treatment-as-usual control group, showed significantly lower rates of substance use at 2-month follow-up – indicating MBRP helps prevent relapses[21]. Similar results were noted in a subsequent study[22].

Depression is also common in these paitents[23]. Marefat and group studied 24 drug addicted individuals, 12 in experimental group who received 60 min thrice weekly yoga sessions for 5 weeks, and 12 in wait list control group. As compared to controls, the individuals in the experimental group had significant decrease in anxiety and depression over the course of the follow-up period[24].

Conclusion

Yoga can help in addiction disorders.

References

1. ASAM: http://www.asam.org/quality-practice/definition-of-addiction (accessed February 5, 2017.
2. World Health Organization (WHO), Global Health Observatory (GHO) [8/31/2012]; Available at: http://www.who.int/gho/substance_abuse/en/index.html.- accessed 1/15/18.
3. Center for Behavioral Health Statistics and Quality. (2016). Key substance use and mental health indicators in the United States: Results from the 2015 National Survey on Drug Use and Health (HHS Publication No.SMA 16-4984, NSDUH Series H-51.
4. Rudd RA, Seth P, David F, Scholl L. Increases in Drug and Opioid-Involved Overdose Deaths — United States, 2010–2015. MMWR Morb Mortal Wkly Rep 2016;65:1445–1452. DOI: dx.doi.org/10.15585/mmwr.mm655051e1.
5. Douaihy AB, Kelly TM, Sullivan C. Medications for substance use disorders. Soc Work Public Health. 2013;28(3-4):264-78. doi: 10.1080/19371918.2013.759031.
6. Klein JW. Pharmacotherapy for Substance Use Disorders. Med Clin North Am. 2016 Jul;100(4):891-910. doi: 10.1016/j.mcna.2016.03.011. Epub 2016 Apr 20.
7. https://www.drugabuse.gov/publications/principles-drug-addiction-treatment-research-based-guide-third-edition/frequently-asked-questions/what-drug-addiction-treatment - accessed 1/16/18.
8. Brandon TH, Vidrine JI, Litvin EB. Relapse and relapse prevention. Annu Rev Clin Psychol. 2007;3:257–284.
9. Hohmann L, Bradt J, Stegemann T, Koelsch S. Effects of music therapy and music-based interventions in the treatment of substance use disorders: A systematic review. Zhang Q, ed. PLoS ONE. 2017;12(11): e0187363. doi:10.1371/ journal.pone. 0187363.
10. Sarkar S, Varshney M. Yoga and substance use disorders: A narrative review. Asian J Psychiatr. 2017 Feb;25:191-196. doi: 10.1016/j.ajp.2016.10.021. Epub 2016 Nov 5.

11. Bock BC, Fava JL, Gaskins R, et al. Yoga as a Complementary Treatment for Smoking Cessation in Women. Journal of Women's Health. 2012;21(2):240-248. doi:10.1089/jwh.2011.2963.

12. L Carim Todd, S Mitchell, B Oken. Does yoga improve smoking cessation outcomes? A systematic review of the literature. BMC Complement Altern Med. 2012; 12(Suppl 1): P389. Published online 2012 Jun 12.

13. Brewer JA, Mallik S, Babuscio TA, et al. Mindfulness training for smoking cessation: results from a randomized controlled trial. Drug Alcohol Depend. 2011;119(1-2):72–80.

14. Hallgren, M., Romberg, K., Bakshi, A.-S., and Andréasson, S. Yoga as an adjunct treatment for alcohol dependence: a pilot study. Complement. Ther. Med. 2014; 22: 441–445.

15. Reddy S, Dick AM, Gerber MR, Mitchell K. The Effect of a Yoga Intervention on Alcohol and Drug Abuse Risk in Veteran and Civilian Women with Posttraumatic Stress Disorder. Journal of Alternative and Complementary Medicine. 2014;20(10):750-756. doi:10.1089/acm.2014.0014.

16. Shaffer HJ, LaSalvia TA, Stein JP. Comparing Hatha yoga with dynamic group psychotherapy for enhancing methadone maintenance treatment: a randomized clinical trial. Altern Ther Health Med. 1997 Jul;3(4):57-66.

17. Zhuang, S., An, S., and Zhao, Y. Yoga effects on mood and quality of life in Chinese women undergoing heroin detoxification: a randomized controlled trial. Nurs. Res. 2013; 62: 260–268.

18. Devi, N.J., Singh, T.B., and Subramanya, P. Effect of yoga on depression and quality of life in drug abusers. Int. J. Ayurveda Pharma Res. 2014; 2: 61–66.

19. Dhawan, A., Chopra, A., Jain, R., Yadav, D., and Vedamurthachar. Effectiveness of yogic breathing intervention on quality of life of opioid dependent users. (null)Int. J. Yoga. 2015; 8: 144–147.

20. Khalsa, S.B.S., Khalsa, G.S., Khalsa, H.K., and Khalsa, M.K. Evaluation of a residential Kundalini yoga lifestyle pilot program for addiction in India. J. Ethn. Subst. Abuse. 2008; 7: 67–79.DOI: dx.doi.org/10.1080/15332640802081968.

21. Witkiewitz K, Bowen S. Depression, craving, and substance use following a randomized trial of mindfulness-based relapse prevention. J Consult Clin Psychol. 2010;78(3):362–74.

22. Khanna S, Greeson JM. A Narrative Review of Yoga and Mindfulness as Complementary Therapies for Addiction. Complementary therapies in medicine. 2013;21(3):244-252. doi:10.1016/j.ctim.2013.01.008.

23. Kodl MM, Fu SS, Willenbring ML, Gravely A, Nelson DB, Joseph AM. The impact of depressive symptoms on alcohol and cigarette consumption following treatment for alcohol and nicotine dependence. Alcoholism: Clinical and Experimental Research. 2008;32:92–99.

24. Marefat, M., Peymanzad, H., and Alikhajeh, Y. The study of the effects of yoga exercises on addicts' depression and anxiety in rehabilitation period. Procedia-Soc. Behav. Sci. 2011; 30: 1494–1498.

Duchenne Muscular Dystrophy

Duchenne muscular dystrophy (DMD) is a genetic disorder characterized by progressive muscle degeneration and weakness[1]. It is one of nine types of muscular dystrophy. DMD is caused by a lack of dystrophin, a protein that helps keep muscle cells intact[2]. Symptom onset is in early childhood, usually between ages 3 and 5[3]. DMD has an X-linked recessive inheritance pattern and the mother is the carrier. The disease primarily affects boys, but in rare cases it can affect girls. It occurs in approximately 1 in 3500 to 5000 live male births. It affects around one in 3,500–5,000 males born worldwide[4]. Muscle weakness can begin as early as age 3, first affecting the muscles of the hips, pelvic area, thighs and shoulders, and later the skeletal (voluntary) muscles in the arms, legs and trunk. The calves are often enlarged. By the early teens, the heart and respiratory muscles also are affected. DMD patients typically lose ambulation in their teenage years and premature fatality often occurs in the third decade of life due to respiratory and cardiac complications[5,6]. The diagnosis can be made after careful review of the history and a good physical examination. The affected boys usually present with developmental delay, proximal weakness, and elevated serum creatine kinase. A muscle biopsy or genetic testing confirms the diagnosis. Due to advances in cardiac and respiratory care, life expectancy of these patients has increased. Affected males can now look forward to attending college, have careers, get married and have children. Survival into the 40s and 50s are known to occur. Traditional treatment has relied mainly on corticosteroids[7].

On Sept. 19, 2016, the U.S. Food and Drug Administration granted accelerated approval to eteplirsen (brand name Exondys 51) as the first disease-modifying drug for DMD. This drug helps promote dystrophin production[8]. The FDA on Feb. 9, 2017, approved deflazacort (brand name Emflaza) to treat DMD. It is a corticosteroid that works by decreasing inflammation and reducing the activity of the immune system in these patients. Complementary and alternative medicine modalities are frequently used by patients and their caregivers for the management of this disease[9]. Yoga has also been used[10].

Yoga and Duchenne Muscular Dystrophy

In a study of 76 patients with DMD, researchers found that only 26 were able to finish the study. These patients were taught hatha yoga breathing exercises and were instructed to perform the exercises three times a day for 10 months. At the end of the study, it was noted that yogic breathing exercises resulted in a significant increase in forced vital capacity and forced expiratory volume in the first second[11].

Conclusion

Yogic breathing exercises may benefit the respiratory functions in patients with DMD, but attrition rate is high.

References

1. Duchenne and Becker muscular dystrophy. Genetics Home Reference (GHR). 2016; ghr.nlm.nih.gov/condition/duchenne-and-becker-muscular-dystrophy – accessed 12/2/17.
2. Hoffman EP, Brown RH, Kunkel LM. Dystrophin: The protein product of the Duchenne muscular dystrophy locus. Cell. 1987;51:919–928.
3. Darras BT, Miller DT, Urion DK. Dystrophinopathies. GeneReviews®. November 26, 2014; ncbi.nlm.nih.gov/books/NBK1119 – accessed 12/2/17.
4. Mendell JR, Shilling C, Leslie ND, et al. Evidence-based path to newborn screening for Duchenne muscular dystrophy. Ann Neurol. 2012;71(3):304–313.
5. D'Orsogna L, O'Shea JP, Miller G. Cardiomyopathy of Duchenne muscular dystrophy. Pediatr Cardiol. 1988;9:205–213.
6. Dittrich S, Tuerk M, Haaker G, Greim V, Buchholz A, Burkhardt B, Fujak A, Trollmann R, Schmid A, Schroeder R. Cardiomyopathy in duchenne muscular dystrophy: current value of clinical, electrophysiological and imaging findings in children and teenagers. Klin Padiatr. 2015;227:225–231.
7. Moxley RT, Ashwal S, Pandya S, et al. Quality Standards Subcommittee of the American Academy of Neurology. Practice Committee of the Child Neurology Society Practice parameter: corticosteroid treatment of Duchenne dystrophy: report of the quality standards subcommittee of the American Academy of Neurology and the practice committee of the Child Neurology Society. Neurology. 2005;64(1):13–20.
8. Ervasti JM. Dystrophin, its interactions with other proteins, and implications for muscular dystrophy. Biochim Biophys Acta. 2007;1772(2):108–117.
9. Zhu Y, Romitti PA, Conway KM, et al. Complementary and Alternative Medicine for Duchenne and Becker Muscular Dystrophies:

Characteristics of Users and Caregivers. Pediatric neurology. 2014;51(1):71-77. doi:10.1016/ j.pediatrneurol.2014.02.003.

10. Telles S, Balkrishna A, Maharana K. Effect of Yoga and Ayurveda on Duchenne Muscular Dystrophy. Indian Journal of Palliative Care. 2011;17(2):169-170. doi:10.4103/0973-1075.84544.

11. Marcos Rojo Rodrigues, Celso Ricardo Fernandes Carvalho, Danilo Forghieri Santaella, Geraldo Lorenzi-Filho, Suely Kazue Nagahashi Marie. Effects of yoga breathing exercises on pulmonary function in patients with Duchenne muscular dystrophy: an exploratory analysis. J Bras Pneumol. 2014 Mar-Apr; 40(2).

Eating Disorders

The Diagnostic and Statistical Manual of Mental Disorders, Fifth Edition, includes the following eating disorders: Anorexia Nervosa, Bulimia Nervosa, Binge Eating Disorder and Feeding or Eating Disorder-Not Elsewhere Classified. The last group consists of Atypical Anorexia Nervosa, Subthreshold Bulimia Nervosa, Subthreshold Binge Eating Disorder and Purging disorder[1].

It is estimated that 13% of young women meet criteria for eating disorders[2]. The prevalence in adolescent and young adult populations in the United States, is as follows: between 0.3 and 0.9 % are diagnosed with anorexia nervosa, between 0.5 and 5 % with bulimia nervosa, between 1.6 and 3.5 % with binge eating disorder, and about 4.8 % with eating disorder otherwise not specified[3-6].

Eating disorders are associated with many co-morbid conditions[7] and carry an increased risk of mortality[8,9]. Many affected individuals have co-morbid psychiatric disorders, including depressive symptoms and anxiety disorders[10]. These patients also have a high rate of suicide[11]. Eating disorders are often accompanied with low confidence and self-esteem, shame and other psychological problems[12-14]. Recurrent vomiting and excessive laxative use can result in dental erosion, esophageal tears, and other medical problems[15].

Unfortunately, less than 25% of individuals with this disorder receive treatment[16]. Remission is difficult, despite treatment[17].

Yoga and Eating Disorders

Many medical clinicians and researchers have recognized the beneficial effect of regular yoga practice in eating disorders[18,19]. Two thirds of the eighteen-inpatient eating disorder treatment programs in the USA, included yoga in their therapeutic regimen, in 2016[20].

Body dissatisfaction and disordered eating behaviors are closely linked[21]. This attitude is changed by yoga[22]. Several well-designed studies have shown that women who do yoga note improvements in both body satisfaction, self-acceptance and disordered eating[23-25]. Co-morbid depression and anxiety are common in patients with eating disorders[26]. In one study, 20 adolescent girls with eating disorders, aged 14–18 years, were enrolled in a 12-week yoga program. At the end of the study, the researchers noted decreases in depression, anxiety, and disordered thoughts about eating[27].

In a study of 38 individuals with eating disorders were randomized into a control group and a yoga group. All were members of a residential eating disorder treatment program. The yoga group did 1 hour of yoga before dinner for 5 days. The yoga group significantly reduced pre-meal negative affect (a desired effect) compared to treatment as usual[28].

Carei and associates studied a total of 50 girls and 4 boys aged 11-21 years with eating disorders (anorexia nervosa, bulimia nervosa, eating disorder not otherwise specified). They were randomized to an 8-week trial of standard care (n=27) vs. individualized yoga plus standard care (n=26). After 12 weeks, the yoga group demonstrated greater decreases in eating disorder symptoms[29].

A randomized trial was conducted with 90 participants (yoga=45; control=45) with binge eating disorder. Participants in the yoga group, underwent 12 weeks of yoga practice. At the end of the study, the researchers found statistically significant self-reported reductions in binge eating and increases in physical activity. There were also statistically significant reductions for body mass index and hips and waist measurement in the yoga group[30].

A review of data from 20 personal journals of 25 women with obesity, revealed that yoga was responsible for a positive shift in eating habits in these women, with an overall reduction in the quantity of food they consumed, decreased eating speed, and an improvement in food choices[31].

Conclusion

Yoga plays an important role in improving body satisfaction in women. Its practice has repeatedly demonstrated an improvement in eating disorders. Yoga practice should be incorporated in all programs designed to help people with these conditions[32].

References

1. Diagnostic and Statistical Manual of Mental Disorders, 5th Edition (DSM-5) American Psychiatric Association, 2013.
2. Stice E, Marti N, Rohde P. Prevalence, incidence, impairment, and course of the proposed DSM-5 eating disorder diagnoses in an 8-year prospective community study of young women. J Abnormal Psychol. in press.
3. Le Grange D, Swanson SA, Crow SJ, Merikangas KR. Eating disorder not otherwise specified presentation in the US population. Int J Eat Disord. 2012;45:711–8. doi: 10.1002/eat.22006.
4. Hudson J, Hiripi E, Pope H, Kessler R. The prevalence and correlates of eating disorders in the National Comorbidity Survey Replication. Biol Psychiatry. 2007;61:348–58. doi: 10.1016/j.biopsych.2006.03.040.
5. Rosen DS. Identification and management of eating disorders in children and adolescents. Pediatr. 2010;126:1240–53. doi: 10.1542/peds.2010-2821.
6. Swanson SA, Crow SJ, LeGrange D, Swendsen J, Merikangas KR. Prevalence and correlates of eating disorders in adolescents: results from the National Comorbidity Survey Replication Adolescent Supplement. Arch Gen Psych. 2011;68:714–23. doi: 10.1001/archgenpsychiatry.2011.22.
7. Mehler P.S., Andersen A.E. Eating Disorders: A Guide to Medical Care and Complications. Johns Hopkins University; Baltimore, MD, USA: 2010.
8. Franko D.L., Keshaviah A., Eddy K.T., Krishna M., Davis M.C., Keel P.K., Herzog D.B. A longitudinal investigation of mortality in anorexia nervosa and bulimia nervosa. Am. J. Psychiatry. 2013;170:917–925. doi: 10.1176/appi.ajp.2013.12070868.
9. Crow S.J., Peterson C.B., Swanson S.A., Raymond N.C., Specker S., Eckert E.D., Mitchell J.E. Increased mortality in bulimia nervosa and other eating disorders. Am. J. Psychiatry. 2009;166:1342–1346.
10. Blinder B, Cumella E, Sanathara V. Psychiatric comorbidities of female inpatients with eating disorders. Psychosom Med. 2006;68(3):454–446. doi: 10.1097/01.psy.0000221254.77675.f5.
11. Bulik CM, Thornton L, Pinheiro AP, Plotnicov K, Klump KL, Brandt H, Crawford S, Fichter MM, Halmi KA, Johnson C, Kaplan AS, Mitchell J, Nutzinger D, Strober M, Treasure J, Woodside DB, Berrettini WH, Kaye WH. Suicide attempts in anorexia nervosa. Psychosom Med. 2008;70(3):378–383.
12. Stice E, Killen JD, Hayward C, Taylor CB. Support for the continuity hypothesis of bulimic pathology. J Consult Clin Psychol. 1998;66(5):784–790.
13. Taylor CB, Altman T, Shisslak C, Bryson S, Estes LS, Gray N, McKnight KM, Kraemer HC, Killen JD. Factors associated with weight concerns in adolescents. Int J Eat Disorders. 1998;24:31–42.
14. Killen JD, Hayward C, Wilson DM, Taylor CB, Hammer LD, Litt I, Simmonds B, Haydel F. Factors associated with eating disorder

symptoms in a community sample of 11- and 12-year-old girls. Int J Eat Disorders. 1994;15:357–3679–11.

15. Mitchell JE, Myers TC, Glass JB. Pharmacotherapy and medical complications of eating disorders in children and adolescents. Child Adolesc Psychiatr Clin N Am. 2002;11(2):365–385.

16. Johnson JG, Cohen P, Kasen S, Brook JS. Eating disorders during adolescence and the risk for physical and mental disorders during early adulthood. Archives of General Psychiatry. 2002;59:545–552.

17. Agras WS, Walsh BT, Fairburn CG, Wilson GT, Kraemer HC. A multicenter comparison of cognitive-behavioral therapy and interpersonal psychotherapy for bulimia nervosa. Archives of General Psychiatry. 2000;57:459–466.

18. Douglass L. Yoga as an intervention in the treatment of eating disorders: Does it help? Eating Disorders. 2009;17(2):126–139.; Douglass L. Thinking through the body: The conceptualization of yoga as therapy for individuals with eating disorders. Eating Disorders. 2011;19(1):83–96.

19. Mehling WE, Wrubel J, Daubenmier JJ, et al. Body Awareness: a phenomenological inquiry into the common ground of mind-body therapies. Philosophy, Ethics, and Humanities in Medicine□: PEHM. 2011;6:6. doi:10.1186/1747-5341-6-6.

20. Frisch M. J., Herzog D. B., Franko D. L. Residential treatment for eating disorders. International Journal of Eating Disorders. 2006;39(5):434–442.

21. Neumark-Sztainer D, Croll J, Story M, Hannan PJ, French S, Perry C. Ethnic/racial differences in weight-related concerns and behaviors among adolescent girls and boys: Findings from Project EAT. J Psychosom Res. 2002;53:963–974.

22. Wyer K. Mirror image: Yoga classes at the Monte Nido clinic are changing how women with eating disorders see themselves. Yoga Journal. 2001;158:70–73.

23. Daubenmier J. The relationship of Yoga, body awareness, and body responsiveness to self-objectification and disordered eating. Psychology of Women Quarterly. 2005;29(2005):207–219.

24. Mitchell K. S., Mazzeo S. E., Rausch S. M., Cooke K. L. Innovative interventions for disordered eating: Evaluating dissonance-based and yoga interventions. International Journal of Eating Disorders. 2007;40(2):120–128. doi: 10.1002/eat.20282.

25. Dittmann K. A., Freedman M. R. Body awareness, eating attitudes, and spiritual beliefs of women practicing yoga. Eating Disorders. 2009;17(4):273–292.

26. Blinder B, Cumella E, Sanathara V. Psychiatric comorbidities of female inpatients with eating disorders. Psychosom Med. 2006;68(3):454–446. doi: 10.1097/01.psy.0000221254.77675.f5.

27. Hall A, Ofei-Tenkorang NA, Machan JT, Gordon CM. Use of yoga in outpatient eating disorder treatment: a pilot study. Journal of Eating Disorders. 2016;4:38. doi:10.1186/s40337-016-0130-2.

28. Pacanowski CR, Diers L, Crosby RD, Neumark-Sztainer D. Yoga in the treatment of eating disorders within a residential program: A randomized controlled trial. Eat Disord. 2017 Jan-Feb;25(1):37-51. Epub 2016 Oct 10.

29. Carei T. R., Fyfe-Johnson A. L., Breuner C. C., Brown M. A. Randomized controlled clinical trial of yoga in the treatment of eating disorders. Journal of Adolescent Health. 2010;46(4):346–351. doi: 10.1016/j.jadohealth.2009.08.007.

30. McIver S, O'Halloran P, McGartland M. Yoga as a treatment for binge eating disorder: a preliminary study. Complement Ther Med. 2009 Aug;17(4):196-202. doi: 10.1016/j.ctim.2009.05.002. Epub 2009 Jun 13.

31. McIver S., McGartland M., O'Halloran P. 'Overeating is not about the food': women describe their experience of a yoga treatment program for binge eating. Qualitative Health Research. 2009;19(9):1234–1245. doi: 10.1177/1049732309343954.

32. Neumark-Sztainer D. Yoga and eating disorders: is there a place for yoga in the prevention and treatment of eating disorders and disordered eating behaviours? Advances in Eating Disorders. 2014;2(2):136-145. doi:10.1080/21662630.2013.862369.

Epilepsy

The International League Against Epilepsy describes epilepsy as, "a disorder of the brain characterized by an enduring predisposition to generate epileptic seizures and by the neurobiological, cognitive, psychological, and social consequences of this condition. The definition of epilepsy requires the occurrence of at least one epileptic seizure"[1]. The transient attack results from an abnormally excessive or synchronous neuronal activity in the brain. Epilepsy is not uncommon – after migraine, stroke and Alzheimer's disease, it is the 4th common neurological problem seen in the US[2]. According to the Centers for Disease Control and Prevention, in 2015, there were about 3.4 million people who suffered from epilepsy (3 million adults and 400,000 children) in the US[3]. Worldwide, approximately 50 million people suffer from epilepsy[4]. There are 3 major groups of seizures – generalized onset seizures, focal onset seizures and unknown onset seizures. Causes are numerous and include congenital conditions, brain damage from perinatal injuries, severe brain trauma, stroke, infections of the brain and brain tumors. In some instances, the cause is never defined.

Treatment with anti-epilepsy drug is cheap and effective. However, it is often complicated by comorbid medical conditions and social obstacles. Co-morbid conditions, like cardiovascular, pulmonary[5] and mental health disorders[6] are often seen in these patients. Epileptic patients also suffer from considerable stigma and social disadvantage[7]. Yoga practice has been beneficial in patients with epilepsy[8].

Yoga and Epilepsy

A twice daily yoga meditation protocol in 20 subjects with drug-resistant epilepsy resulted in a decrease in the frequency of seizures in 19 of the 20 participants. The reductions were noted within the first three months. Yoga was performed for three months. In six patients, there was a more than 50% reduction in the seizure frequency[9].

In another study, the investigators found that yoga therapy was able to reduce seizures by 57% in a group of patients with epilepsy[10].

In a trial of 18 drug resistant patients with EEG confirmed epilepsy, yoga reduced the frequency of seizures. Patients also reported an improvement in their quality of life[11].

In another study of 32 patients with idiopathic epilepsy, Sahaja Yoga practice for 6 months resulted in an 86% decrease in seizure frequency[12]. Improvements in EEG with yoga in drug resistant epilepsy patients was also reported by another group of researches[13].

Meditation was performed for one year by 11 refractory epilepsy patients. The meditation group not only showed a decrease in frequency and duration of seizures after 6 months of yoga practice but also demonstrated normalization of the EEG[14].

Using the Beck Anxiety Inventory, Tang and associates found significant reductions in anxiety scores in patients with epilepsy, with meditation intervention. The benefit was also confirmed by a significant reduction in anxiety in the yoga intervention group using McNemar tests[15]. Mindfulness based interventions also improve the quality of life of these patients, especially those with associated depression[16].

A recent Cochrane review confirmed a possible beneficial effect of yoga in the control of seizures[17].

Conclusion

Yoga appears to be beneficial in epilepsy. Stress is often a precipitating factor in seizure activity – yoga induces relaxation and therefore reduces stress.

References

1. Fisher RS; van Emde Boas W; Blume W; Elger C; Genton P; Lee P; Engel J. Epileptic seizures and epilepsy: definitions proposed by the International League Against Epilepsy (ILAE) and the International Bureau for Epilepsy (IBE). Epilepsia. 2005; 46(4):470-2.
2. https://www.epilepsy.com/learn/about-epilepsy-basics/epilepsy-statistics - accessed 12/16/17.

3. Zack MM, Kobau R. National and state estimates of the numbers of adults and children with active epilepsy — United States, 2015. MMWR. 2017;66:821–825.

4. http://www.who.int/mediacentre/factsheets/fs999/en/ - accessed 12/18/17.

5. Centers for Disease Control and Prevention Comorbidity in adults with epilepsy—United States, 2010. MMWR Surveill Summ. 2013;62:849–53.

6. Tellez-Zenteno JF, Patten SB, Jetté N, Williams J, Wiebe S. Psychiatric comorbidity in epilepsy: a population-based analysis. Epilepsia. 2007;48:2336–44.

7. Centers for Disease Control and Prevention (CDC) Epilepsy surveillance among adults—19 states, Behavioral Risk Factor Surveillance System, 2005. MMWR. 2008;57:1–20.

8. Yardi N. Yoga for control of epilepsy. Seizure. 2001;10:7–12.

9. Rajesh B, Jayachandran D, Mohandas G, Radhakrishnan K. A pilot study of a yoga meditation protocol for patients with medically refractory epilepsy. J Altern Complement Med. 2006;12:367–71.

10. Sirven JI, Drazkowski JF, Zimmerman RS, Bortz JJ, Shulman DL, Macleish M. Complementary/alternative medicine for epilepsy in Arizona. Neurology. 2003;61:576–7.

11. Lundgren T, Dahl J, Yardi N, Melin L. Acceptance and Commitment Therapy and yoga for drug-refractory epilepsy: A randomized controlled trial. Epilepsy Behav. 2008;13:102–8.

12. Panjwani, U., Selvamurthy, W., Singh, S. H., Gupta, H. L., Thakur, L. and Rai, U. C. Effect of Sahaja Yoga practice on seizure control and EEG changes in patients of epilepsy. Indian Journal of Medical Research 1996; 103: 165–172.

13. D Deepak, K. K., Manchanda, S. K. and Maheshwari, M. C. Meditation improves clinicoelectroencephalographic measures in drug resistant epileptics. Biofeedback and Selfregulation 1994; 19: 25–40.

14. Ramaratnam S, Sridharan K. Cochrane review. Cochrane epilepsy group Ti: Yoga for epilepsy SO: The Cochrane database of systematic review. 2006.

15. Tang V, Poon WS, Kwan P. Mindfulness-based therapy for drug-resistant epilepsy: an assessor-blinded randomized trial. Neurology. 2015;85(13):1100–7.

16. Thompson NJ, Walker ER, Obolensky N, Winning A, Barmon C, DiIorio C, Compton MT. Distance delivery of mindfulness-based cognitive therapy for depression: project UPLIFT. Epilepsy Behav. 2010;19(3):247–54.

17. Panebianco M, Sridharan K, Ramaratnam S. Yoga for epilepsy. Cochrane Database Syst Rev. 2017 Oct 5;10:CD001524.

Fibromyalgia

Fibromyalgia is debilitating condition. It is characterized by widespread musculo-skeletal pain, and is often accompanied by fatigue, memory problems, and sleep disturbances[1]. The musculo-skeletal discomfort is characterized by chronic diffuse aches, stiffness and soft tissue tenderness.

Some studies suggest that it may affect 2%–8% of the adult population[2]. It is more common in women and is the most common cause of generalized, musculoskeletal pain in women between the ages of 20 and 55 years[3]. In the US, it is estimated to affect 11-15 million people[4].

Fibromyalgia is often associated with one or more of several sensitivity conditions, such as chronic fatigue syndrome, irritable bowel syndrome, myofascial pain syndrome, restless leg syndrome, and interstitial cystitis/bladder pain syndrome[5]. Diagnosis is usually made using the 2010 American College of Rheumatology self-report questionnaire (the Fibromyalgia Survey Questionnaire), which is primarily based on patient symptoms[6]. A score of ≥12 has a 93.1% sensitivity and 91.7% specificity for this disease[1]. The pathophysiology is multifactorial, and includes dysfunction of the CNS pain modulatory systems, dysfunction of the neuroendocrine system, and dysautonomia[7].

Treatment is usually multicomponent and is directed at improving pain, fatigue, depression, and quality of life. Pregabalin has been approved by the FDA to treat fibromyalgia and helps reduce pain sensation[8,9]. Other common medications used include pain relievers such as acetaminophen and NSAIDs. Antidepressants such as duloxetine and milnacipran also help ameliorate the pain and fatigue in these patients[10]. They also help improve the depressed mood, sleep disturbances, and decreased quality of life experienced by these patients. Amitriptyline[11] or cyclobenzaprine[12] may also be given to relieve insomnia and other symptoms. Other medication often used is gabapentin. However, the FDA approved therapies are only 30% effective in relieving symptoms and only 20% effective in improving function[13]. Many of these drugs have significant side effects and are often too expensive for many patients[14].

Physical and occupational therapy is also helpful in these patients[15]. Cognitive behavioral techniques have shown some benefit[16]. Several nutritional supplements, such as CoQ10 and l-carnitine have also shown some benefit in these patients[17,18]. Yoga has also been studied for its therapeutic benefits in patients with fibromyalgia[19].

Yoga and Fibromyalgia

Carson and associates found that yoga practice in 53 women with fibromyalgia improved pain, fatigue, stiffness, sleep problems, tenderness, balance, vigor, and strength. They also noted an improvement in accompanying psychological conditions such as depression, anxiety, cognition deficits, and coping with and reacting to emotionally negative situations (confrontation, self-isolation, disengagement, and catastrophizing). The researchers also noted that more practice of yoga was associated with a greater relief in patients with firbromyalgia[20].

In another study, a combination of yoga/Tui Na (Chinese massage therapy) and yoga alone was studied in 40 women with fibromyalgia. Both groups reported (Fibromyalgia Impact Questionnaire) benefit after 8 weeks[21].

In a study of 22 fibromyalgia patients, yoga was given twice weekly for 8 weeks. Each class was 75 minutes in duration. The researchers found that symptoms of continuous pain, pain catastrophizing and pain acceptance improved significantly in these patients with yoga practice. Serum cortisol levels were also improved[22].

In a small study of 11 patients, Hennard found significant improvement in stiffness, anxiety, and depression, in patients with fibromyalgia. A better quality of life was also reported[23].

In a more recent study, gentle Hatha yoga reduced fibromyalgia-related symptoms, as recorded in the Fibromyalgia Impact Questionnaires provided by the participants and evaluation of manual tender points. The study involved 10 patients with fibromyalgia, aged 39-64 years. Yoga was given 2 times a week for 8 weeks[24].

Stress reduction techniques also offer benefit for these patients[25]. Yoga is a good stress reliever[26].

A meta-analysis of yoga and other complementary and alternative medicine modalities in patients with fibromyalgia revealed no severe adverse effects[27].

Conclusion

Yoga appears to help decrease some of the symptoms in patients with fibromyalgia.

References

1. Clauw DJ. (2014) Fibromyalgia: a clinical review. JAMA 311:1547–1555.
2. Branco JC, Bannwarth B, Failde I, Abello Carbonell J, Blotman F, Spaeth M, Saraiva F, Nacci F, Thomas E, Caubère JP, et al. (2010) Prevalence of fibromyalgia: a survey in five European countries. Semin Arthritis Rheum 39:448–453.
3. Branco JC, Bannwarth B, Failde I, Abello Carbonell J, Blotman F, Spaeth M, Saraiva F, Nacci F, Thomas E, Caubère JP, et al. (2010) Prevalence of fibromyalgia: a survey in five European countries. Semin Arthritis Rheum 39:448–453.
4. White KP, Harth M. Classification, epidemiology, and natural history of fibromyalgia. Curr Pain Headache Rep. 2001;5:320–9.
5. Yunus MB. (2007) Fibromyalgia and overlapping disorders: the unifying concept of central sensitivity syndromes. Semin Arthritis Rheum 36:339–356.
6. Wolfe F, Clauw DJ, Fitzcharles MA, Goldenberg DL, Häuser W, Katz RS, Mease P, Russell AS, Russell IJ, Winfield JB. (2011) Fibromyalgia criteria and severity scales for clinical and epidemiological studies: a modification of the ACR Preliminary Diagnostic Criteria for Fibromyalgia. J Rheumatol 38:1113–1122.
7. Lawson K. Treatment options and patient perspectives in the management of fibromyalgia: Future trends. Neuropsychiatr Dis Treat. 2008;4:1059–71.
8. Häuser W, Petzke F, Üçeyler N, Sommer C. (2011) Comparative efficacy and acceptability of amitriptyline, duloxetine and milnacipran in fibromyalgia syndrome: a systematic review with meta-analysis. Rheumatology (Oxford) 50:532–543.

9. Häuser W, Bernardy K, Uçeyler N, Sommer C. (2009c) Treatment of fibromyalgia syndrome with gabapentin and pregabalin—a meta-analysis of randomized controlled trials. Pain 145:69–81.
10. Häuser W, Bernardy K, Uçeyler N, Sommer C. (2009b) Treatment of fibromyalgia syndrome with antidepressants: a meta-analysis. JAMA 301:198–209.
11. Clemons A, Vasiadi M, Kempuraj D, Kourelis T, Vandoros G, Theoharides TC. (2011) Amitriptyline and prochlorperazine inhibit proinflammatory mediator release from human mast cells: possible relevance to chronic fatigue syndrome. J Clin Psychopharmacol 31:385–387.
12. Moldofsky H, Harris HW, Archambault WT, Kwong T, Lederman S. (2011) Effects of bedtime very low dose cyclobenzaprine on symptoms and sleep physiology in patients with fibromyalgia syndrome: a double-blind randomized placebo-controlled study. J Rheumatol 38:2653–2663.
13. Russell IJ, Mease PJ, Smith TR, Kajdasz DK, Wohlreich MM, Detke MJ, Walker DJ, Chappell AS, Arnold LM. Efficacy and safety of duloxetine for treatment of fibromyalgia in patients with or without major depressive disorder: results from a 6-month, randomized, double-blind, placebo-controlled, fixed-dose trial. Pain. 2008;136:432–44.
14. Mease PJ, Choy EH. Pharmacotherapy of fibromyalgia. Rheumatic Diseases Clinics of North America. 2009;35(2):359–372. doi: 10.1016/j.rdc.2009.06.007.
15. Offenbächer M, Stucki G. Physical therapy in the treatment of fibromyalgia. Scand J Rheumatol Suppl. 2000;113:78-85.
16. Bernardy K, Füber N, Köllner V, Häuser W. (2010) Efficacy of cognitive-behavioral therapies in fibromyalgia syndrome - a systematic review and meta-analysis of randomized controlled trials. J Rheumatol 37:1991–2005.
17. Cordero MD, Cano-García FJ, Alcocer-Gómez E, De Miguel M, Sánchez-Alcázar JA. (2012a) Oxidative stress correlates with headache symptoms in fibromyalgia: coenzyme Q_{10} effect on clinical improvement. PLoS One 7:e35677.
18. Rossini M, Di MO, Valentini G, Bianchi G, Biasi G, Cacace E, Malesci D, La MG, Viapiana O, Adami S. (2007) Double-blind, multicenter trial comparing acetyl l-carnitine with placebo in the treatment of fibromyalgia patients. Clin Exp Rheumatol 25:182–188.
19. Carson JW, Carson KM, Jones KD, Bennett RM, Wright CL, Mist SD. A pilot randomized controlled trial of the Yoga of Awareness program in the management of fibromyalgia. Pain. 2010;151:530–9.
20. Carson JW, Carson KM, Jones KD, Mist SD, Bennett RM. Follow-up of Yoga of Awareness for Fibromyalgia: Results at 3 Months and Replication in the Wait-list Group. The Clinical journal of pain. 2012;28(9):804-813.
21. Da Silva GD, Lorenzi-Filho G, Lage LV. Effects of yoga and the addition of Tui Na in Patients with Fibromyalgia. J Altern Complement Med. 2007;13:1107–14.

22. Curtis K, Osadchuk A, Katz J. An eight-week yoga intervention is associated with improvements in pain, psychological functioning and mindfulness, and changes in cortisol levels in women with fibromyalgia. Journal of Pain Research. 2011;4:189-201. doi:10.2147/JPR.S22761.
23. Hennard J. A protocol and pilot study for managing fibromyalgia with yoga and meditation. Int J Yoga Therapy. 2011;(21):109–121.
24. Rudrud L. Gentle Hatha yoga and reduction of fibromyalgia-related symptoms: a preliminary report. Int J Yoga Therap. 2012;(22):53–57.
25. Goldenberg DL, Kaplan KH, Nadeau MG, Brodeur C, Smith S, Schmid CH. A controlled study of a stress-reduction, cognitive-behavioral treatment program in fibromyalgia. Journal of Musculoskeletal Pain. 1994;2:53–66.
26. Vempati R. P., Telles S. (2000). Baseline occupational stress levels and physiological responses to a two day stress management program. J. Indian Psychol. 18, 33–37.
27. Mist SD, Firestone KA, Jones KD. Complementary and alternative exercise for fibromyalgia: a meta-analysis. Journal of Pain Research. 2013;6:247-260. doi:10.2147/JPR.S32297.

Gastroesophageal Reflux Disease (GERD)

Gastroesophageal reflux disease (GERD) is common in the USA, affecting about 18%-28% of the population[1]. It is also common in other parts of the world[2]. Typical symptoms of GERD are heartburn, regurgitation, and epigastric pain. Pharmacologic treatment usually consists of an 8-week course with either a proton pump inhibitor (PPI) or an H2 receptor blocker[3]. Surgical intervention is sometimes required, especially if the patient is non-responsive to medications or if there are complications. Frequent or severe symptoms result in an impaired health-related quality of life[4]. It is also a risk factor for adenocarcinoma of the esophagus. Lifestyle modifications include losing weight (if overweight), smoking cessation, avoiding alcohol, chocolate, citrus juice, and tomato-based products, avoiding large and spicy meals and waiting 2 to 3 h after a meal before lying down, especially if there are nocturnal symptoms[5]. Over the counter use of anti-GERD medications are common[6]. Complementary and alternative medicine is often used by patients in upper gastro-intestinal (GI) disorders[7].

Yoga and GERD

A case report in one patient with GI reflux, regularly practice of Kapalbhati (A pranayama technique in which inspiration is passive and expiration is active through abdominal muscles) and Agnisar kriya (a method of contracting or "flapping" abdominal muscles in and out to promote improved digestion and gastrointestinal motility) along with PPI, showed improvement. The authors contend that these interventions increased diaphragmatic tone and reduced transient lower esophageal sphincter (LES) relaxation and increased LES tone, thereby helping the GI reflux[8].

Yoga practice also helps in losing weight. It also helps in smoking cessation and alcohol abuse disorder – conditions that are often associated with GERD[9-11].

Conclusion

Yoga may have a therapeutic potential in the complimentary treatment of GERD.

References

1. El-Serag HB, Sweet S, Winchester CC, et al. Update on the epidemiology of gastro-oesophageal reflux disease: a systematic review. Gut. 2013.
2. Nocon M, Labenz J, Willich SN. Lifestyle factors and symptoms of gastro-oesophageal reflux -- a population-based study. Aliment Pharmacol Ther. 2006;23(1):169–74.
3. DeVault K., Castell D. (2005) Updated guidelines for the diagnosis and treatment of gastroesophageal reflux disease. Am J Gastroenterol 100: 190–200.
4. Revicki D., Wood M., Maton P., Sorensen S. (1998) The impact of gastroesophageal reflux disease on health-related quality of life. Am J Med 104: 252–258.
5. Singhal V, Khaitan L. Gastroesophageal Reflux Disease: Diagnosis and Patient Selection. The Indian Journal of Surgery. 2014;76(6):453-460. doi:10.1007/s12262-014-1090-x.
6. Nebel OT, Fornes MF, Castell DO. Symptomatic gastroesophageal reflux: incidence and precipitating factors. Am J Dig Dis. 1976;21(11):953–956. doi: 10.1007/BF01071906.
7. Comar KM, Kirby DF. Herbal Remedies in Gastroenterology. J Clin Gastroenterol. 2005;39:457–468. doi: 10.1097/01.mcg.0000165650.09500.3a.
8. Kaswala D, Shah S, Mishra A, et al. Can yoga be used to treat gastroesophageal reflux disease? International Journal of Yoga. 2013;6(2):131-133. doi:10.4103/0973-6131.113416.
9. Cramer H, Sushila Thoms M, Anheyer D, Lauche R, Dobos G. Yoga in Women With Abdominal Obesity— a Randomized Controlled Trial. Deutsches Ärzteblatt International. 2016;113(39):645-652. doi:10.3238/arztebl.2016.0645.
10. McIver S, O'Halloran P, McGartland M. The impact of Hatha yoga on smoking behavior. Altern Ther Health Med. 2004 Mar-Apr;10(2):22-3.
11. Reddy S, Dick AM, Gerber MR, Mitchell K. The Effect of a Yoga Intervention on Alcohol and Drug Abuse Risk in Veteran and Civilian Women with Posttraumatic Stress Disorder. Journal of Alternative and Complementary Medicine. 2014;20(10):750-756. doi:10.1089/acm.2014.0014.

Hypertension

Hypertension is a common disease[1]. According to the World Health Organization, it affected about 40% of adults aged 25 and over, worldwide, in 2008[2]. It is the main risk factor for the development of coronary heart disease, stroke, heart failure and arterial aneurysm – the main causes of cardiovascular morbidity and mortality[3,4]. Globally, it is responsible for approximately 45% of deaths due to heart disease and 51 % of deaths due to stroke[5]. Hypertension related deaths of about 9.4 million worldwide each year, are expected to rise in the coming years[5].

Even pre-hypertensives (blood pressure between 120/80 mmHg and 139/89 mmHg) experience an increased risk for cardiovascular complications when compared to normotensives[6]. According to the new guidelines[7], prehypertensives are now categorized as elevated or stage I hypertension. The new hypertension guidelines are: Normal: Less than 120/80 mm Hg; Elevated: systolic between 120-129 and diastolic less than 80; Stage 1: systolic between 130-139 or diastolic between 80-89; Stage 2: systolic at least 140 or diastolic at least 90 mm Hg; Hypertensive crisis: systolic over 180 and/or diastolic over 120.

Hypertension is primarily treated with pharmaceuticals[8]. Lifestyle changes (salt and alcohol reduction, calorie restriction and physical exercise) are also included in most guidelines[9], and widely accepted as being beneficial[10]. Despite these measures, a significant number of patients do not reach goal, and are labelled resistant[11].

Resistant hypertension, is present in about 10-15% of all hypertensive patients[12-15]. It is defined as blood pressure that is uncontrolled despite the use of 3 or more antihypertensive agents from different classes or blood pressure controlled with the use 4 or more agents[16]. Patients with resistant hypertension are at a higher risk to develop complications such as stroke, heart disease or congestive heart failure[17,18].

The SPRINT trial suggested a lower treatment goal in hypertensives - reducing systolic blood pressure to 120 mm Hg decreased heart attacks, heart failure and stroke by one third and mortality by a quarter when compared to a goal of 140 mm Hg[19]. Yoga may help reach this lower goal in hypertensives without additional polypharmacy.

Complementary and alternative medicine interventions are also common in use for blood pressure control[20,21]. Yoga positively modulates hypertension and appears to have a feasible role as an adjunct life-style intervention in hypertensive patients[22,23].

Yoga and Hypertension

A reduction in blood pressure (BP) is instrumental in reducing cardiovascular morbidity and mortality[24]. Though the yoga induced reductions may be small, they are like that achieved by other lifestyle modifications advocated by current guidelines[25]. In a meta-analysis of 61 observational studies of BP and mortality (1 million adults) even a small 2 mmHg fall in mean systolic blood pressure was associated with a 7% lower risk of ischemic heart disease death and a 10% lower risk of stroke death[26]. Similarly, a 2 mmHg decrease in diastolic blood pressure reduces the risk of coronary heart disease by 6%, and stroke by 15%[27].

There is a multitude of research studies reporting reductions in both systolic and diastolic blood pressures with the practice of yoga, in normal individuals and in hypertensives, with or without cardiovascular complicatons[28-30]. Favorable results have also been seen in hypertensives with other co-morbid conditions[31].

A randomized controlled trial of 26 patients in the yoga group and 31 patients in the usual care group was done for 12 weeks, with 24-h ambulatory BP monitoring. All patients were yoga naïve and had untreated prehypertension or Stage 1 hypertension. After twelve weeks of yoga, 24 h systolic blood pressure decreased by 6 mmHg, and diastolic blood pressure reduced by 5 mmHg, compared to baseline[32].

Many other trials have confirmed the blood pressure reducing effects of yoga practice. Their presence has allowed several meta-analytic studies to be done.

In a meta-analytic review of 17 studies (22 trials), yoga was associated with a small but clinically significant decline in both systolic and diastolic blood pressure (average: −4.17 and −3.26 mmHg, respectively[33].

Another group included a total of 6 studies (involving 386 patients) in a meta-analytic review. They reported that although the included trials were of poor methodology, there were encouraging decreases in both systolic and diastolic blood pressure in all studies[34]. Blood pressure reducing effects of yoga practice were also reported by another meta-analysis of 10 studies[35].

In a study to review the benefits of meditation, researchers selected 19 eligible studies. In the meta-analysis, they reported that yogic meditation was noted to reduce systolic and diastolic blood pressure by a mean of 4.02 mmHg[36].

Breathing exercises also play a role in decreasing blood pressure. Fifteen minutes of alternate-nostril yoga breathing in fifteen healthy male volunteers significantly decreased systolic blood pressure[37].

Yoga also improves the quality of life in hypertensive patients[38,39].

Conclusion

Yoga practice demonstrates blood pressure reductions in most studies.

References

1. Lim SS, Vos T, Flaxman AD, Danaei G, et al A comparative risk assessment of burden of disease and injury attributable to 67 risk factors and risk factor clusters in 21 regions, 1990-2010 : a systematic analysis for the Global Burden of Disease Study 2010. Lancet. 2012; 380 (9859): 2224-60.
2. http://ish-world.com/downloads/pdf/global_brief_hypertension.pdf - accessed 1/18/18.
3. Sante D. Pierdomenico, Domenico Lapenna, Roberta Di Tommaso, Silvio Di Carlo, Anna L. Esposito, Rocco Di Mascio, Enzo Ballone, Franco Cuccurullo, Andrea Mezzetti. Blood Pressure Variability and Cardiovascular Risk in Treated Hypertensive Patients.American Journal of Hypertension, Volume 19, Issue 10, 1 October 2006,
4. Dorjgochoo T, Shu XO, Zhang X, et al. Relation of blood pressure components and categories and all-cause, stroke and coronary heart disease mortality in urban Chinese women: A population-based

prospective study. Journal of hypertension. 2009;27(3):468-475. doi:10.1097/HJH.0b013e3283220eb9.

5. World Health Organisation. A global brief on hypertension: silent killer, global public health crisis. 2013. http://apps.who.int/iris/bitstream/10665/79059/1/WHO_DCO_WHD_201 3.2_eng.pdf?ua=1. Accessed 12 January 2018.

6. Hsia J, Margolis KL, Eaton CB, Wenger NK, Allison M, Wu L, et al. Prehypertension and cardiovascular disease risk in the Women's Health Initiative. Circulation. 2007;115(7):855–860.

7. Paul K. Whelton, Robert M. Carey, Wilbert S. Aronow et al. 2017 ACC/AHA/AAPA/ABC/ACPM/AGS/APhA/ASH/ASPC/NMA/PCNA Guideline for the Prevention, Detection, Evaluation, and Management of High Blood Pressure in Adults. A Report of the American College of Cardiology/American Heart Association Task Force on Clinical Practice Guidelines. Journal of the American College of Cardiology, November 2017. DOI: 10.1016/j.jacc.2017.11.006.

8. Hackam DG, Khan NA, Hemmelgarn BR, et al. The 2010 Canadian Hypertension Education Program recommendations for the management of hypertension: part 2 - therapy. Can J Cardiol. 2010 May;26(5):249-58.; NIHCG, 2013.

9. Erdine S, Ari O, Zanchetti A, Cifkova R et al. ESH-ESC guidelines for the management of hypertension. Herz. 2006 Jun;31(4):331-8.

10. Nicoll R, Henein MY. Hypertension and lifestyle modification: how useful are the guidelines? The British Journal of General Practice. 2010;60(581):879-880. doi:10.3399/bjgp10X544014.

11. Wanpen Vongpatanasin. Resistant Hypertension.A Review of Diagnosis and Management. JAMA. 2014;311(21):2216-2224.

12. Persell SD. Prevalence of resistant hypertension in the United States, 2003-2008. Hypertension. 2011;57:1076–1080.

13. Egan BM, Zhao Y, Axon RN, Brzezinski WA, Ferdinand KC. Uncontrolled and apparent treatment resistant hypertension in the United States, 1988-2008. Circulation. 2011;124:1046–1058.

14. de la Sierra A, Segura J, Banegas JR, Gorostidi M, de la Cruz JJ, Armario P, Oliveras A, Ruilope LM. Clinical features of 8295 patients with resistant hypertension classified on the basis of ambulatory blood pressure monitoring. Hypertension. 2011;57:898–902.

15. Roberie DR, Elliott WJ. What is the prevalence of resistant hypertension in the United States. Curr Opin Cardiol. 2012;27:386–391.

16. Calhoun DA, Jones D, Textor S, Goff DC, Murphy TP, Toto RD, White A, Cushman WC, White WB, Sica D, Ferdinand K, Giles TD, Falkner B, Carey RM. American Heart Association Scientific statement on resistant hypertension: diagnosis, evaluation, and treatment. Hypertension. 2008;51:1403–1419.

17. Pierdomenico SD, Lapenna D, Bucci A, Di Tommaso R, Di Mascio R, Manente BM, Caldarella MP, Neri M, Cuccurullo F, Mezzettti A. Cardiovascular outcome in treated hypertensive patients with responder, masked, false resistant and true resistant hypertension. Am J Hypertens. 2005;18:1422–1428.

18. Isaksson H, Ostergren J. Prognosis in therapy-resistant hypertension. J Intern Med. 1994;236:643–649.

19. NIH 2015: http://www.nhlbi.nih.gov/news/press-releases/2015/landmark-nih-study-shows-intensive-blood-pressure-management-may-save-lives. Accessed 1/19/18.

20. Osamor PE, Owumi BE. Complementary and alternative medicine in the management of hypertension in an urban Nigerian community. BMC Complementary and Alternative Medicine. 2010;10:36. doi:10.1186/1472-6882-10-36.

21. Wang J, Xiong X. Evidence-Based Chinese Medicine for Hypertension. Evidence-based Complementary and Alternative Medicine□: eCAM. 2013;2013:978398. doi:10.1155/2013/978398.

22. Cohen D, Townsend RR. Yoga and hypertension. The Journal of Clinical Hypertension. 2007;9:800–801.

23. Wolff M, Sundquist K, Larsson Lönn S, Midlöv P. Impact of yoga on blood pressure and quality of life in patients with hypertension – a controlled trial in primary care, matched for systolic blood pressure. BMC Cardiovascular Disorders. 2013;13:111. doi:10.1186/1471-2261-13-111.

24. Bangalore S, Gong Y, Cooper-DeHoff RM, et al. 2014 Eighth Joint National Committee panel recommendation for blood pressure targets revisited: results from the INVEST study. J Am Coll Cardiol. 2014 Aug 26;64(8):784-93.

25. Subramanian H., M. B. Soudarssanane, R. Jayalakshmy, et al., "Non-pharmacological interventions in hypertension: a community-based cross-over randomized controlled trial," Indian Journal of Community Medicine, vol. 36, pp. 191–196, 2011.

26. Lewington S, Clarke R, Qizilbash N, Peto R, Collins R. Age-specific relevance of usual blood pressure to vascular mortality: a meta-analysis of individual data for one million adults in 61 prospective studies. The Lancet. 2002;360(9349):1903–1913.

27. Cook NR, Cohen J, Hebert PR, et al. Implications of small reductions in diastolic blood pressure for primary prevention. Arch Intern Med. 1995;155(7):701–709.

28. Shirley Telles, Sadhana Verma, Sachin Kumar Sharma, Ram Kumar Gupta, and Acharya Balkrishna. Alternate-Nostril Yoga Breathing Reduced Blood Pressure While Increasing Performance in a Vigilance Test. Med Sci Monit Basic Res. 2017; 23: 392–398. doi: 10.12659/MSMBR.906502.

29. Cohen DL, Bloedon LT, Rothman RL, et al. Iyengar Yoga versus Enhanced Usual Care on Blood Pressure in Patients with Prehypertension to Stage I Hypertension: A Randomized Controlled Trial. Evidence-based Complementary and Alternative Medicine: eCAM. 2011;2011:546428. doi:10.1093/ecam/nep130.

30. Hartley L, Dyakova M, Holmes J. et al. Yoga for the primary prevention of cardiovascular disease. Cochrane Database Syst Rev. 2014 May 13;5:CD010072.

31. Cade T, Reeds DN, Mondy KE, et al. Yoga lifestyle intervention reduces blood pressure in HIV-infected adults with cardiovascular disease risk factors. HIV medicine. 2010;11(6):379-388. doi:10.1111/j.1468-1293.2009.00801.x.

32. Cohen DL, Bloedon LT, Rothman RL, et al. Iyengar Yoga versus Enhanced Usual Care on Blood Pressure in Patients with Prehypertension to Stage I Hypertension: A Randomized Controlled Trial. Evidence-based Complementary and Alternative Medicine: eCAM. 2011;2011:546428. doi:10.1093/ecam/nep130.

33. Hagins M, States R, Selfe T, et al. Effectiveness of Yoga for Hypertension: Systematic Review and Meta-Analysis Evidence-Based Complementary and Alternative Medicine. Volume 2013 (2013), Article ID 649836, 13 pages.

34. Wang J, Xiong X, Liu W (2013) Yoga for Essential Hypertension: A Systematic Review. PLoS ONE 8(10): e76357. https://doi.org/10.1371/journal.pone.0076357

35. Okonta Nkechi. Does yoga therapy reduce blood pressure in patients with hypertension? An integrative review. Holist Nurs Pract 2012; 26: 137-141.; Tyagi A, Cohen M. Yoga and hypertension: a systematic review. Altern Ther Health Med. 2014 Mar-Apr;20(2):32-59.

36. Yang H, Wu X, Wang M. The Effect of Three Different Meditation Exercises on Hypertension: A Network Meta-Analysis. Evidence-based Complementary and Alternative Medicine: eCAM. 2017;2017:9784271. doi:10.1155/2017/9784271.

37. Shirley Telles, Sadhana Verma, Sachin Kumar Sharma, Ram Kumar Gupta, and Acharya Balkrishna. Alternate-Nostril Yoga Breathing Reduced Blood Pressure While Increasing Performance in a Vigilance Test. Med Sci Monit Basic Res. 2017; 23: 392–398. doi: 10.12659/MSMBR.906502.

38. Wolff M, Sundquist K, Larsson Lönn S, et al. Impact of yoga on blood pressure and quality of life in patients with hypertension - a controlled trial in primary care, matched for systolic blood pressure. BMC Cardiovasc Disord. 2013 Dec 7;13: 111.

39. Wolff M, Ashfaque A. Memon, John P, et al. Yoga's effect on inflammatory biomarkers and metabolic risk factors in a high-risk population - a controlled trial in primary care. BMC Cardiovasc Disord. 2015 Aug 19; 15:91.

Human Immunodeficiency Virus/Acquired Immune Deficiency Syndrome (HIV/AIDS)

There were an estimated 37,600 new HIV infections in 2014[1]. Most of these infections (70%) occur in gay and bisexual men, with 23% occurring in heterosexual individuals and the remaining 7% among people who inject drugs[2]. According to the Centers for Disease Control and Prevention, there were about 1,122,900 adults and adolescents who were living with HIV at the end of 2015, with 162,500 (15%) of these, remaining undiagnosed. HIV was responsible for 6,721 deaths in 2014. Worldwide, it is estimated that there were approximately 36.7 million people (2.1 million of these were children less than 15 years old) living with HIV/AIDS at the end of 2016[3]. Almost 30% of HIV infected people did not know their HIV status (in 2016)[4]. Half the infected individuals are women[5].

HIV infected patients may have no symptoms in the beginning but as the disease progresses, the immune system worsens, and signs and symptoms of various infections become apparent. Besides flu like illness, there may be swollen lymph nodes, weight loss, fever, diarrhea and cough. Serological tests, such as rapid diagnostic tests or enzyme immunoassays, are commonly used for diagnosis. They detect the presence or absence of antibodies to HIV-1/2 and/or HIV p24 antigen. Treatment is usually given according to the 2016 World Health Organization (WHO) treatment guidelines[6]. With increased awareness and the introduction of antiretroviral treatment regimens, the infection and death rate from HIV infections has been falling. According to WHO, HIV infections fell by 39% and HIV related deaths fell by one third between the years 2000 and 2016[7].

Yoga and HIV/AIDS

Use of complementary and alternative medicine (CAM) is prevalent among HIV+ individuals[8]. Published data indicates that 60% of these individuals use CAM to treat HIV-related health concerns[9,10].

HIV infected patients are at an increased risk of cardiovascular disease[11]. Yoga may help prevent against the increased cardio-metabolic risk faced by HIV infected patients. In a study of 60 HIV infected patients, 20 weeks of supervised yoga practice reduced both the systolic and diastolic pressure when compared to patients in the control standard treatment group[12].

HIV infected patients have a poor quality of life[13]. Breathing exercises as prescribed in the Sudarshan Kriya yoga (a comprehensive breathing and relaxation technique) were given to a randomized yoga group. Of the 61 patients in the study (31 in the yoga group and 30 in the control group), researchers noted that using the WHOQOL-HIVBREF questionnaire[14], patients in the yoga group reported significant improvement in the quality of their life[15]. Patients with HIV infection often suffer from stress, anxiety, substance abuse and depression[16-18], conditions that are improved with Sudarshan Kriya Yoga[19].

Several studies have indicated that mindfulness-based stress reduction (MBSR) may help patients with HIV infection[20-22]. Antiretroviral therapies are often associated with side effects[23]. MBSR has demonstrated benefit in reducing the frequency of symptoms attributable to these drugs, at three and six months post intervention, compared to the waitlist group[24].

Conclusion

Yoga practice shows potential in improving the quality of life of HIV/AIDS patients.

References

1. https://www.cdc.gov/hiv/statistics/overview/ataglance.html accessed 12/1/17.
2. Singh S et al. (CDC). HIV incidence, prevalence, and undiagnosed infections in men who have sex with men. Presentation at Conference on Retroviruses and Opportunistic Infections, 2017, Seattle, WA.
3. http://www.unaids.org/en/resources/fact-sheet- 1/3/18 accessed.
4. http://www.unaids.org/en/resources/fact-sheet-accessed 1/3/18.
5. WHO. HIV/AIDS 2015 [Internet] [cited 2015 Aug 1]. Available from: http://www.who.int/mediacentre/factsheets/fs360/en/- accessed 11/19/17.
6. http://www.who.int/hiv/mediacentre/en/- accessed 1/4/18.
7. http://www.who.int/mediacentre/factsheets/fs360/en/-accessed 1/4/18.
8. Littlewood RA, Vanable PA. Complementary and Alternative Medicine Use Among HIV+ People: Research Synthesis and Implications for HIV

Care. AIDS care. 2008;20(8):1002-1018.
doi:10.1080/09540120701767216.

9. Duggan J, Peterson WS, Schutz M, Khuder S, Charkraborty J. Use of
    complementary and alternative therapies in HIV-infected patients. AIDS
    Patient Care and STDs. 2001;15(3):159–167.

10. Mikhail IS, DiClemente R, Person S, Davies S, Elliott E, Wingood G, et
    al. Association of complementary and alternative medicines with HIV
    clinical disease among a cohort of women living with HIV/AIDS. Journal
    of Acquired Immune Deficiency Syndrome. 2004;37(3):1415–1422.

11. Grinspoon SK, Grunfeld C, Kotler DP, et al. State of the Science
    Conference. Initiative to decrease cardiovascular risk and increase
    quality of care for patients living with HIV/AIDS executive summary.
    Circulation. 2008;118:198–210.

12. Cade T, Reeds DN, Mondy KE, et al. Yoga lifestyle intervention reduces
    blood pressure in HIV-infected adults with cardiovascular disease risk
    factors. HIV medicine. 2010;11(6):379-388. doi:10.1111/j.1468-
    1293.2009.00801.x.

13. Mahalakshmy T, Premarajan K, Hamide A. Quality of life and its
    determinants in people living with human immunodeficiency virus
    infection in Puducherry, India. Indian J Community Med. 2011;36:203–
    7.

14. Skevington SM, Lotfy M, O'Connell KA WHOQOL Group. The World
    Health Organization's WHOQOL-BREF quality of life assessment:
    Psychometric properties and results of the international field trial. A
    report from the WHOQOL group. Qual Life Res. 2004;13:299–310.

15. Mawar N, Katendra T, Bagul R, et al. Sudarshan Kriya yoga improves
    quality of life in healthy people living with HIV (PLHIV): results from an
    open label randomized clinical trial. The Indian Journal of Medical
    Research. 2015;141(1):90-99.

16. Byrd DA, Fellows RP, Morgello S, et al. Neurocognitive Impact of
    Substance Use in HIV Infection. Journal of acquired immune deficiency
    syndromes (1999). 2011;58(2):154-162.
    doi:10.1097/QAI.0b013e318229ba41.

17. Rosenfield BD. Pain in ambulatory AIDS patients: impact of pain on
    psychology functioning and quality of life. Pain 1996;68:323–328.

18. Leserman J, Petitto JM, Perkins DO, Folds JD, Golden RN, Evans DL.
    Severe stress, depressive symptoms, and changes in lymphocyte
    subsets in human immunodeficiency virus-infected men. A 2-year
    follow-up study. Archives of General Psychiatry. 1997;54(3):279–85

19. Zope SA, Zope RA. Sudarshan kriya yoga: breathing for health. Int J
    Yoga. 2013;6:4–10.

20. logsdon-Conradsen S. Using mindfulness meditation to promote holistic
    health in individuals with HIV/AIDS. Cognitive and Behavioral Practice.
    2002;9(1):67–72.

21. Barrows K. The application of mindfulness to HIV. Focus. 2006;21(8):1–
    8.

22. SeyedAlinaghi S, Jam S, Foroughi M, et al. RCT of Mindfulness-Based
    Stress Reduction Delivered to HIV+ Patients in Iran: Effects on CD4+ T

Lymphocyte Count and Medical and Psychological Symptoms. Psychosomatic Medicine. 2012;74(6):620-627. doi:10.1097/PSY.0b013e31825abfaa.

23. Johnson MO, Charlebois E, Morin SF, et al. Perceived adverse effects of antiretroviral therapy. J Pain Symptom Manage. 2005;29:193–205.

24. Duncan LG, Moskowitz JT, Neilands TB, Dilworth SE, Hecht FM, Johnson MO. Mindfulness-Based Stress Reduction for HIV Treatment Side Effects: A Randomized Wait-List Controlled Trial. Journal of Pain and Symptom Management. 2012;43(2):161-171. doi:10.1016/j.jpainsymman.2011.04.007.

Infertility

Infertility is defined as not being able to get pregnant (conceive) after one year (or longer) of unprotected sex[1]. It is estimated that 6% of married women aged 15 to 44 years (in the USA) are unable to get pregnant despite trying for one year or more. It is estimated that about 12% of women aged 15 to 44 years, regardless of their marital status, are also unable to get pregnant after one year of trying. According to the Centers for Disease Control and Prevention, about 12% of women aged 15 to 44 years (in the USA) have difficulty getting pregnant or carrying a pregnancy to term, regardless of their marital status. It is estimated that infertility affects 8-10% of couples worldwide, and 7-15% of couples in United States[2].

Men are responsible for this problem in about 35% of cases. Male infertility may be due to several causes and these include: varicoceles, trauma to the testes, certain medications and supplements, certain cancer treatments, and several medical conditions and hormonal disorders. Medical treatments that can reduce a man's fertility include diabetes, cystic fibrosis, certain types of autoimmune disorders, and certain types of infections. Hormonal disorders include diseases of the hypothalamus or pituitary glands. Rarely genetic conditions such as Klinefelter's syndrome, Y-chromosome microdeletion, myotonic dystrophy, and some less common genetic disorders[1]. Infertility is also reduced by lifestyle factors in men, including aging, smoking, excessive alcohol use, being obese, marijuana use, exposure to testosterone and radiation, frequent exposure of the testes to high temperatures, exposure to certain medications such as flutamide, cyproterone, bicalutamide, spironolactone, ketoconazole, or cimetidine, and exposure to environmental toxins including pesticides, lead, cadmium, or mercury[1]. In women, causes of infertility include polycystic ovarian syndrome, diminished ovarian reserve, functional hypothalamic amenorrhea, improper function of the hypothalamus and pituitary glands, premature ovarian insufficiency, menopause and fallopian tube obstruction, and an anatomically abnormal uterus[3]. Infertility is further aggravated by many lifestyle factors in women, including aging, smoking, excessive alcohol use, extreme weight gain or loss and excessive physical or emotional stress that results in amenorrhea (absent periods)[1]. Male infertility is treated with medical, surgical, or assisted reproductive therapies depending on the underlying cause. In women, treatment may include medications (clomiphene, letrozole, human menopausal gonadotropin, follicle stimulating hormone, gonadotropin-releasing hormone, metformin and bromocriptine) and artificial insemination. Yoga may play a beneficial role in the treatment of infertility[3,4].

Yoga and Infertility

Women with infertility are often anxious[5]. In a study involving twelve weeks of holistic yoga, ninety adolescent (15-18 years) girls with polycystic ovarian syndrome noticed a significant improvement in anxiety when compared to a regular exercise program[6].

Infertility treatments, especially in vitro fertilization (IVF), induce significant stress in women. The shavasana yoga pose, done for 10 minutes every day for 4 weeks, has been shown to induce physiological changes consistent with reduction of stress[7]. Relaxation with yoga has shown to be helpful in ameliorating the psychological distress in women undergoing IVF treatment[8]. In another study involving 49 infertile women, a 6-week yoga class, was instrumental in reducing anxiety and depression. There was also an improvement in fertility-specific quality of life while these women were waiting for IVF[9]. Stress in these women may alter the biochemistry in a way that it is not conducive to conception[10]. Relaxation may therefore improve a women's treatment results, and this has been substantiated[11].

Stress and anxiety in the men of infertile couples may also play a role in reduced conception[12]. Yoga practices are very efficacious in reducing stress and anxiety[13]. The yoga technique of 'moola bandha' stimulates the pelvic floor area, increasing awareness and improving sexual desire and functioning in people[14].

The beneficial effects of yoga practices in pregnant women have been highlighted by Sengupta[15]. Yoga practiced by pregnant women 1 h daily resulted in an increase in birth weight, decrease in preterm labor, with no increase in complications[16].

Conclusion

Yoga practice may be beneficial in the reduction of infertility.

References

1. https://www.cdc.gov/reproductivehealth/infertility/index.htm - accessed 11/19/17.
2. Centers for disease control and prevention. Infertility (Data for the U.S.) [Last accessed on July 18, 2012]. Available from: http://www.cdc.gov/nchs/fastats/fertile.htm .
3. Khalsa HK. Yoga: an adjunct to infertility treatment. Fertil Steril. 2003 Oct;80 Suppl 4:46-51.
4. Darbandi S, Darbandi M, Khorram Khorshid HR, Sadeghi MR. Yoga Can Improve Assisted Reproduction Technology Outcomes in Couples with Infertility. Altern Ther Health Med. 2017 Nov 7. pii: AT5482.
5. Mansson M, Holte J, Landin-Wilhelmsen K, Dahlgren E, Johansson A, Landon M. Women with polycystic ovary syndrome are often depressed or anxious-a case control study. Psychoneuroendocrinology. 2008;33:1132–8.
6. Nidhi R, Padmalatha V, Nagarathna R, Amritanshu R. Effect of holistic yoga program on anxiety symptoms in adolescent girls with polycystic ovarian syndrome: A randomized control trial. International Journal of Yoga. 2012;5(2):112-117. doi:10.4103/0973-6131.98223.
7. Sharma G, Mahajan K, Sharma L. Shavasana-Relaxation technique to combat stress. Journal of Bodywork and Movement Therapies. 2007;11(2):173–80. doi: 10.1016/j.jbmt.2007.01.002.
8. Nekavand M, Mobini N, Sheikhi A, Roshandel S, Sheikhi A. A survey on the impact of relaxation on anexiety and the result of IVF in patients with infertility that have been referd to the infertility centers of Tehran university of medical sciences during 2012–2013. J Urmia Nurs Midwifery Fac. 2015;13(7):605–12.
9. Oron G., Allnutt E., Lackman T., Sokal-Arnon T., Holzer H., Takefman J. A prospective study using Hatha Yoga for stress reduction among women waiting for IVF treatment. Reproductive BioMedicine Online. 2015;30(5):542–548. doi: 10.1016/j.rbmo.2015.01.011.
10. Csemiczky G, Landgren BM, Collins A. The influence of stress and state anxiety on the outcome of IVF-treatment: Psychological and endocrinological assessment of Swedish women entering IVF-treatment. Acta Obstet Gynecol Scand. 2000;79:113–8.
11. Valiani M, Abedian S, Ahmadi M, Pahlavanzade S. The effects of relaxation on outcome treatment in infertile women. Complementary Medicine Journal of faculty of Nursing & Midwifery. 2014;4(2):845–53.
12. Song S-H, Kim DS, Kim HJ, Kim JW, Ryu SW, Hong JY, et al. Psychological stress and sexual function of male partner of infertile couple during fertile period. Fertil Steril. 2014;102(3) doi: 10.1016/j.fertnstert.2014.07.372.

13. Streeter CC, Whitfield TH, Owen L, et al. Effects of Yoga Versus Walking on Mood, Anxiety, and Brain GABA Levels: A Randomized Controlled MRS Study. Journal of Alternative and Complementary Medicine. 2010;16(11):1145-1152.
14. Sengupta P, Chaudhuri P, Bhattacharya K. Male reproductive health and yoga. International Journal of Yoga. 2013;6(2):87-95. doi:10.4103/0973-6131.113391.
15. Sengupta P. Health impacts of yoga and Pranayama: A state-of-the-art review. Int J Prev Med. 2012;3:444–58.
16. Narendran S, Nagarathna R, Narendran V, Gunasheela S, Nagendra HR. Efficacy of yoga on pregnancy outcome. J Altern Complement Med. 2005;11:237–44.

Insomnia

According to the American Society of Sleep Medicine, insomnia is common. They estimate that 30 to 35% adults have brief symptoms of insomnia. About 15 to 20% have a short-term insomnia disorder (lasting less than three months.) while 10% have a chronic insomnia disorder (occurring at least three times per week for at least three months)[1]. Patients with insomnia usually complain difficulty in going to sleep, awakening after falling asleep, finding it hard to get back to sleep, awakening too early in the morning, or combinations of these problems. Poor sleep leads to a diminished sense of well-being and impaired daytime functioning (depressive or irritable mood, loss in concentration, learning and memory capacities). The diagnosis of insomnia is primarily dependent of the patient's own perception of their sleep. Polysomnography is sometimes used to define the sleep disorder[2]. Poor sleep has been linked to diminished immunity, weight gain, obesity, inflammation, cardiovascular disease, diabetes, and increased mortality[3].

Patients with insomnia often take over the counter sleep agents (such as melatonin). Prescription drugs commonly used to treat insomnia include safer benzodiazepines and hypnotics - zolpidem, zopiclone and zaleplon. However, long-term use of hypnotic agents can lead to drug tolerance, dependence, or rebound insomnia. Antidepressants, antipsychotics, and anticonvulsants are often prescribed, but are not approved by the U.S. Food and Drug Administration for insomnia. Nonpharmacologic options-- including combinations of behavioral interventions, sleep-restriction therapy, and patient education—are also effective and appear to provide longer-lasting benefits. Exercise has also been prescribed with good response[4].

Yoga and Insomnia

Monitoring sleep-wake diaries, Dr. Khalsa documented improvements in 20 patients after 8 weeks of yoga. The benefit was noted in sleep efficiency, total sleep time, total wake time, sleep onset latency, and wake time after sleep onset[5].

In a study in seniors, 68 residents from a home for the aged were randomly allocated to three groups: yoga (physical postures, relaxation techniques, voluntarily regulated breathing and lectures on yoga philosophy), Ayurveda (herbal preparations), and wait-list control (no intervention). After six months, the yoga group showed significant improvement – they slept faster, slept longer and felt more rested in the morning. The other groups showed no significant change[6]. In another study of seniors, 128 individuals aged 60 and older, yoga resulted in improved sleep quality, decreased depression, and better health status[7]. In a subsequent study, 55 seniors were given 6 months of yoga exercises. At the end of the study, the participants reported significant improved sleep quality. They also noted a reduction in depression, sleep disturbances and daytime dysfunction[8]. Yoga intervention has also shown an improvement in sleep quality in women with hot flashes[9] and osteoarthritis[10].

Yoga has also been shown to help cancer survivors sleep better. In one study, 410 survivors of cancer underwent pranayama (breathing exercises), 16 gentle Hatha and restorative yoga asanas (postures), and meditation, in two 75-minute sessions per week. The researchers found that participants in the yoga program demonstrated greater improvements in global sleep quality and, secondarily, subjective sleep quality, daytime dysfunction, sleep efficiency, and medication use post-intervention, compared with standard care participants[11]. Several other studies have also reported an improvement in insomnia in cancer patients with yoga practice[12-16].

Mindfulness meditation when combined with other cognitive behavior therapy in 30 participants resulted in statistically and clinically significant improvements in several nighttime symptoms of insomnia[17].

Conclusion

Studies indicate that yoga practice helps patients sleep better, even when insomnia is due to other medical disorders.

References

1. http://www.sleepeducation.org/news/2014/03/10/insomnia-awareness-day-facts-and-stats - accessed 11/15/17.
2. Littner M, Hirshkowitz M, Kramer M, Kapen S, Anderson WM, et al. Practice parameters for using polysomnography to evaluate insomnia: an update. Sleep. 2003;26:754–60.
3. Grandner MA, Alfonso-Miller P, Fernandez-Mendoza J, Shetty S, Shenoy S, Combs D. Sleep: Important Considerations for the Prevention of Cardiovascular Disease. Current opinion in cardiology. 2016;31(5):551-565.
4. Yang PY, Ho KH, Chen HC, et al. Exercise training improves sleep quality in middle-aged and older adults with sleep problems: A systematic review. J Physiother. 2012;58:157–163.
5. Khalsa SB. Treatment of chronic insomnia with yoga: a preliminary study with sleep-wake diaries. Appl Psychophysiol Biofeedback. 2004 Dec;29(4):269–78.
6. Manjunath NK, Telles S. Influence of Yoga and Ayurveda on self-rated sleep in a geriatric population. Indian J Med Res. 2005 May;121(5):683–90.
7. Chen KM, Chen MH, Chao HC, Hung HM, Lin HS, Li CH. Sleep quality, depression state, and health status of older adults after silver yoga exercises: cluster randomized trial. Int J Nurs Stud. 2009;46(2):154–163.
8. Chen KM, Chen MH, Lin MH, Fan JT, Lin HS, Li CH. Effects of yoga on sleep quality and depression in elders in assisted living facilities. J Nurs Res. 18(1):53–61.
9. Booth-LaForce C, Thurston RC, Taylor MR. A pilot study of a Hatha yoga treatment for menopausal symptoms. Maturitas. 2007;57(3):286–295.
10. Taibi DM, Vitiello MV. A pilot study of gentle yoga for sleep disturbance in women with osteoarthritis. Sleep medicine. 2011;12(5):512-517. doi:10.1016/j.sleep.2010.09.016.
11. Mustian KM, Sprod LK, Janelsins M, et al. Multicenter, Randomized Controlled Trial of Yoga for Sleep Quality Among Cancer Survivors. Journal of Clinical Oncology. 2013;31(26):3233-3241. doi:10.1200/JCO.2012.43.7707.
12. Bower JE, Garet D, Sternlieb B, et al. Yoga for persistent fatigue in breast cancer survivors: A randomized controlled trial. Cancer. 2011.
13. Carson JW, Carson KM, Porter LS, Keefe FJ, Seewaldt VL. Yoga of Awareness program for menopausal symptoms in breast cancer survivors: results from a randomized trial. Supportive care in cancer: official journal of the Multinational Association of Supportive Care in Cancer. 2009;17:1301–9.
14. Ulger O, Yagl NV. Effects of yoga on the quality of life in cancer patients Complement. Ther Clin Pract. 2010;16:60–3.

15. Vadiraja SH, Rao MR, Nagendra RH, et al. Effects of yoga on symptom management in breast cancer patients: A randomized controlled trial. International journal of yoga. 2009;2:73–9.
16. Mustian KM, Janelsins M, Peppone LJ, Kamen C. Yoga for the Treatment of Insomnia among Cancer Patients: Evidence, Mechanisms of Action, and Clinical Recommendations. Oncology & hematology review. 2014;10(2):164-168.
17. Ong J, Shapiro S, Manbar R. Combining mindfulness meditation with cognitive-behavior therapy for insomnia: a treatment development study. Behav Ther. 2008;39(2):171–182.

Interstitial Cystitis/Bladder Pain Syndrome

Interstitial cystitis/bladder pain syndrome is different from bacterial cystitis. Interstitial cystitis is characterized by daytime and nighttime urinary frequency, urgency, and pelvic pain. The symptoms last for more than 6 months and no clear cause is identified. The American Urological Association describes it as "An unpleasant sensation (pain, pressure, discomfort) perceived to be related to the urinary bladder, associated with lower urinary tract symptoms of more than six weeks duration, in the absence of infection or other identifiable causes"[1]. It is more common in females and it is estimated that it may affect up to 11% of women[2]. It is often underdiagnosed. Available treatments are difficult and discontinuation rates are as high as 80%[3]. Therapy consists of supportive, behavioral, and pharmacologic measures. There is no effective long-term treatment available[4]. Surgical intervention is rarely indicated. Complimentary treatments have been tried in these patients[5,6]. Yoga has also been tried[7].

Yoga and Interstitial Cystitis/Bladder Pain Syndrome

No studies could be found using traditional yoga asanas or pranayama in these patients. One study looked at mindfulness based stress reduction (MBSR) in this syndrome with positive results.

Women were randomized to usual care (n=11) or to usual care plus an 8-week MBSR class (n=9). Questionnaires completed at baseline and post-treatment included the O'Leary-Sant Symptom Problem Index, visual analog pain scale, Short Form Health Survey, Female Sexual Function Index, and Pain Self-Efficacy Questionnaire. The Global Response Assessment was completed post-treatment. At the end of the treatment, more MBSR participants' symptoms were improved on the GRA. This group also showed greater improvement in OSPI total and problem scores and Pain Self-Efficacy Questionnaire scores. O'Leary-Sant Symptom Problem Index symptom score change did not differ. Pain Self-Efficacy Questionnaire scores improved in MBSR compared to usual care. Female Sexual Function Index change was similar in both groups. The authors reported that eighty-six percent of MBSR participants felt more empowered to control symptoms. All patients in the MBSR group indicated a desire to continue this adjunct treatment[8].

Conclusion

One study using MBSR demonstrated benefit in patients with interstitial cystitis/bladder pain syndrome .

References

1. Hanno PM, Burks DA, Clemens JQ, Dmochowski RR, Erickson D, Fitzgerald MP, Forrest JB, Gordon B, Gray M, Mayer RD, Newman D, Nyberg L, Jr, Payne CK, Wesselmann U, Faraday MM. AUA guideline for the diagnosis and treatment of interstitial cystitis/bladder pain syndrome. The Journal of urology. 2011;185(6):2162–2170. doi: 10.1016/j.juro.2011.03.064.
2. Clemens JQ, Meenan RT, O'Keeffe Rosetti MC, Brown SO, Gao SY, Calhoun EA. Prevalence of interstitial cystitis symptoms in a managed care population. The Journal of urology. 2005;174(2):576–580.
3. Hanno PM, Burks DA, Clemens JQ, Dmochowski RR, Erickson D, Fitzgerald MP, Forrest JB, Gordon B, Gray M, Mayer RD, Newman D, Nyberg L, Jr, Payne CK, Wesselmann U, Faraday MM. AUA guideline for the diagnosis and treatment of interstitial cystitis/bladder pain syndrome. The Journal of urology. 2011;185(6):2162–2170. doi: 10.1016/j.juro.2011.03.064.
4. Ogawa T, Ishizuka O, Ueda T, Tyagi P, Chancellor MB, Yoshimura N. Current and emerging drugs for interstitial cystitis/bladder pain syndrome (IC/BPS). Expert Opin Emerg Drugs. 2015;20(4):555-70. doi: 10.1517/14728214.2015.1105216. Epub 2015 Nov 4.
5. O'Hare PG, 3rd, Hoffmann AR, Allen P, Gordon B, Salin L, Whitmore K. Interstitial cystitis patients' use and rating of complementary and alternative medicine therapies. International urogynecology journal. 2013;24(6):977–982. doi: 10.1007/s00192-012-1966-x.
6. Atchley MD, Shah NM, Whitmore KE. Complementary and alternative medical therapies for interstitial cystitis: an update from the United States. Translational Andrology and Urology. 2015;4(6):662-667. doi:10.3978/j.issn.2223-4683.2015.08.08.
7. Glickman-Simon R, Ehrlich A. Omega-3 supplementation and cardiovascular disease, acupuncture and chronic obstructive pulmonary disease (COPD), myofascial physical therapy and interstitial cystitis, and yoga and chronic pain. Explore (NY). 2013 Jan-Feb;9(1):54-7. doi: 10.1016/j.explore.2012.11.006.
8. Kanter G, Komesu YM, Qaedan F, et al. Mindfulness-Based Stress Reduction as a Novel Treatment for Interstitial Cystitis/Bladder Pain Syndrome: A Randomized Controlled Trial. International urogynecology journal. 2016;27 (11):1705-1711. doi:10.1007/s00192-016-3022-8.

Irritable Bowel Syndrome

Irritable bowel syndrome (IBS) has an estimated global prevalence of 11.2%[1]. It is a functional multifactorial disease. It is often associated with other functional disorders of the upper and lower gastrointestinal (GI) system[2], and functional non-gastrointestinal syndromes, such as urological chronic pelvic pain syndrome, overactive bladder, prostatic pain syndrome, premenstrual syndrome, sexual (including erectile) dysfunction, fibromyalgia syndrome, chronic fatigue syndrome, migraine, eating disorders, and others[3]. Some psychiatric conditions such as anxiety and depression are also common in these patients[4]. Patients with IBS also report a poor quality of life[5].

IBS is more common in females[6]. Diagnosis is based on symptoms[7]. Most patients complain of abdominal pain and/or discomfort associated with an abnormal bowel habit – diarrhea or constipation or both. The presence of these symptoms for ≥3 days per month in the past 3 months, with symptom onset ≥6 months before, is usually diagnostic of IBS[8]. Most clinicians also rule out other organic diseases, before diagnosing this syndrome[9]. Treatment is usually aimed at symptoms, and includes antispasmodics for abdominal pain, laxatives for constipation and anti-diarrhea medications for diarrhea[10]. Low dose anti-depressants are sometimes used[11]. Foods that aggravate the symptoms are avoided[12]. A non-absorbable antibiotic, rifaximin, and probiotics are sometimes used to alter the GI bacteria[13,14]. Patients not responding to drugs for a year are advised to undergo cognitive–behavioral therapy, hypnotherapy (gut-directed hypnosis) or other psychological therapy, such as psychodynamic (interpersonal) therapy[15].

Yoga and Irritable Bowel Syndrome

The use of complementary and alternative medicine is common in patients with IBS[16]. Yoga has shown benefits in the management of IBS[17,18].

A total of 51 participants completed a two-month Iyengar Yoga intervention (yoga = 29; usual-care waitlist = 22). The classes of 1.5 hours duration were held twice a week. The adolescent (14-17 years) yoga group reported significantly improved physical functioning, and the young adults (18–26 years) yoga group reported significantly improved IBS symptoms (disability, psychological distress, sleep quality, and fatigue) when compared to the control group[19].

Yoga therapy is also effective in young children, ages 8-18. Researchers recorded significant decrease in pain frequency in 20 children after 10 yoga classes. The pain decrease persisted after 3 months, especially in the 8-11 age group[20].

Psychological symptoms are also improved in patients with IBS with yoga therapy. Twenty-five adolescents aged 11 to 18 years with IBS, randomly assigned to either a yoga or wait list control group, were given a one-hour instructional session, demonstration and practice, followed by four weeks of daily home practice guided by a video. After four weeks, adolescents in the yoga group reported improved functional status, decreased emotion-focused avoidance and lower anxiety following the intervention than adolescents in the control group[21].

A Cochrane review of six randomized controlled trials with a total of 273 patients led the authors to suggest that yoga might be a feasible and safe adjunctive treatment for people with IBS[22].

Conclusion

Yoga therapy appears to be beneficial in relieving some of the symptoms of IBS, especially in children and adolescents.

References

1. Enck P, Aziz Q, Barbara G, et al. Irritable bowel syndrome. Nature reviews Disease primers. 2016;2:16014. doi:10.1038/nrdp.2016.14.
2. Ford AC, Forman D, Bailey AG, Axon AT, Moayyedi P. Irritable bowel syndrome: a 10-yr natural history of symptoms and factors that influence consultation behavior. Am. J. Gastroenterol. 2008;103:1229–1239.
3. Whitehead WE, et al. Comorbidity in irritable bowel syndrome. Am. J. Gastroenterol. 2007;102:2767–2776.
4. Janssens KA, Zijlema WL, Joustra ML, Rosmalen JG. Mood and anxiety disorders in chronic fatigue syndrome, fibromyalgia, and irritable bowel syndrome: results from the LifeLines Cohort study. Psychosom. Med. 2015;77:449–457.

5. Gralnek IM, Hays RD, Kilbourne A, Naliboff B, Mayer EA. The impact of irritable bowel syndrome on health-related quality of life. Gastroenterology. 2000;119:654–660.
6. Lovell RM, Ford AC. Effect of gender on prevalence of irritable bowel syndrome in the community: systematic review and meta-analysis. Am. J. Gastroenterol. 2012;107:991–1000.
7. (Longstreth GF, et al. Functional bowel disorders. Gastroenterology. 2006;130:1480–1491.
8. Longstreth GF, et al. Functional bowel disorders. Gastroenterology. 2006;130:1480–1491.
9. Spiegel BM, Farid M, Esrailian E, Talley J, Chang L. Is irritable bowel syndrome a diagnosis of exclusion?: A survey of primary care providers, gastroenterologists, and IBS experts. Am. J. Gastroenterol. 2010;105:848–858.
10. Enck P, Aziz Q, Barbara G, et al. Irritable bowel syndrome. Nature reviews Disease primers. 2016;2:16014. doi:10.1038/nrdp.2016.14.
11. National Institute of Health and Care Excellence. CG61 Irritable bowel syndrome in adults: diagnosis and management of irritable bowel syndrome in primary care. NICE. 2008 [online], http://www.nice.org.uk/guidance/cg61/documents. – accessed 1/5/18.
12. Posserud I, et al. Symptom pattern following a meal challenge test in patients with irritable bowel syndrome and healthy controls. United European Gastroenterol. J. 2013;1:358–367.
13. Pimentel M, et al. Rifaximin therapy for patients with irritable bowel syndrome without constipation. N. Engl. J. Med. 2011;364:22–32.
14. Didari T, Mozaffari S, Nikfar S, Abdollahi M. Effectiveness of probiotics in irritable bowel syndrome: updated systematic review with meta-analysis. World J. Gastroenterol. 2015;21:3072–3084.
15. National Institute of Health and Care Excellence. CG61 Irritable bowel syndrome in adults: diagnosis and management of irritable bowel syndrome in primary care. NICE. 2008 [online], http://www.nice.org.uk/guidance/cg61/documents.- accessed 1/5/18.
16. Hussain Z, Quigley EM. Systematic review: Complementary and alternative medicine in the irritable bowel syndrome. Aliment Pharmacol Ther. 2006;23:465–471.
17. Taneja I, Deepak KK, Poojary G, Acharya IN, Pandey RM, Sharma MP. Yogic versus conventional treatment in diarrhea-predominant irritable bowel syndrome: A randomized control study. Appl Psychophysiol Biofeedback. 2004;29:19–33.
18. Raghavan R, Nielson-Joseph A, Naliboff B, Zeltzer L. The effects of yoga in adolescents with irritable bowel syndrome: A pilot study J Adolesc Health 200026104(Abst).
19. Evans S, Lung KC, Seidman LC, Sternlieb B, Zeltzer LK, Tsao JCI. Iyengar Yoga for Adolescents and Young Adults With Irritable Bowel Syndrome. Journal of pediatric gastroenterology and nutrition. 2014;59(2):244-253.

20. Brands MM, Purperhart H, Deckers-Kocken JM. A pilot study of yoga treatment in children with functional abdominal pain and irritable bowel syndrome. Complement Ther Med. 2011;19:109–114.
21. Kuttner L, Chambers CT, Hardial J, et al. A randomized trial of yoga for adolescents with irritable bowel syndrome. Pain Res Manag. 2006;11:217–223.
22. Schumann D, Anheyer D, Lauche R, Dobos G, Langhorst J, Cramer H. Effect of Yoga in the Therapy of Irritable Bowel Syndrome: A Systematic Review. Clin Gastroenterol Hepatol. 2016 Dec;14(12):1720-1731. doi: 10.1016/j.cgh.2016.04.026. Epub 2016 Apr 22.

Menopausal Disorders

"Menopause" is the permanent cessation of ovulation and menses – the final menstrual period is followed by 12 consecutive months without a menstrual period[1]. Menopause results in a loss of reproductive capacity. It is estimated that 6000 American women aged 40 to 59 years reach menopause daily with a minimum of another 20 years of life expectancy[2]. In the United States, the average age for menopause is 51 years. Menopause, although occurring naturally in most women, is sometimes a result of bilateral oophorectomy (surgical menopause) or chemicals (chemical menopause). Perimenopause is the 3-to-5-year period before menopause and is related to a significant drop in the woman's estrogen levels. The chance of getting pregnant during this period is reduced.

Menopause is often associated with a litany of symptoms. These include, depression, hot flashes, night sweats, sleep disturbances, urinary problems, and vaginal dryness. There may be associated obesity, difficulty in concentrating, thinning of hair, and breast shrinkage[3]. Post-menopausal women are also at an increased risk to develop breast cancer, cardiovascular disease, osteoporosis, and urinary incontinence.

Treatments are numerous and may include hormone replacement, antidepressants, gabapentin, clonidine, and vaginal estrogen. Drug treatment may also be given for osteoporosis. Better nutrition, exercise and psychological interventions are often incorporated in the management.

Yoga and Menopausal Disorders

Booth-LaForce and associates[4] conducted a prospective within-group pilot with 12 peri-menopausal and post-menopausal women experiencing at least 4 menopausal hot flashes per day, and during at least 4 days per week. A 10-week Hatha yoga program resulted in a reduction in total menopausal symptoms, hot-flash daily interference; and improved sleep efficiency in these women.

In another study, one hundred twenty perimenopausal participants (ages 40-55 y) were randomly divided into two study arms: yoga and control. The yoga group practiced for 8 weeks, while the control group did a set of simple physical exercises. (1 h daily, 5 days per week). Assessments made by Greene Climacteric Scale, Perceived Stress Scale, and Eysenck's Personality Inventory before and after the intervention revealed that the yoga group experienced decreases in menopausal symptoms, perceived stress, and neuroticism better than the physical exercise group[5].

In a study of 37 breast cancer survivors complaining of menopause related hot flashes, an 8-week yoga awareness program resulted in marked improvement in symptoms. At eight weeks, they reported a decrease in hot-flash frequency and severity. These improvements persisted at 3 months. They also experienced improvements in joint pains, fatigue, and mood[6].

Yoga was found to be effective in reducing menopausal symptoms in 44 women after 4 months of intervention. These women also noted a reduction in insomnia and an improvement in their quality of life[7].

In a 12-week 3×2 randomized, controlled, factorial design trial, 355 perimenopausal and postmenopausal women, ages 40-62 years, were randomized to yoga (n=107) (90 minutes daily), exercise (n=106) (aerobic exercise 3 times per week), or usual activity (n=142). They were also randomized to a double-blind comparison with ingestion of omega-3 (n=177) (0.615 gram omega-3 supplement, 3 times/day) or placebo (n=178) capsules. After 12 weeks, improvements were seen for Menopausal Quality of Life Questionnaire, vasomotor symptoms and sexuality domain scores in the yoga vs. aerobic exercise group[8].

Improvement in the quality of life were also noted in other studies[9-11]. An improvement in mood and the quality of life was also noted in 164 low active women with 4 months of yoga and physical exercise[12]. Several studies have also noted an improvement in sleep disorders in these pateints[13,14]. Two studies did not find any advantage of yoga practice in reducing hot flashes associated with menopause[15,16].

Cramer and associates in a meta-analysis of 5 randomized control trials, found that yoga intervention was associated with a moderate evidence for short-term effectiveness for psychological symptom relief in menopausal women[17].

Conclusion

Most studies report that yoga practice is helpful in reducing menopausal symptoms, especially hot flashes, mood and sleep disturbances. The quality of life is also improved in these patients.

References

1. World Health Organization (WHO) Research on the Menopause in the 1990s: Report of WHO Scientific Group. Geneva: WHO; 1996.; Harlow BL, Signorello LB. Factors associated with early menopause. Maturitas. 2000;35(1):3–9.
2. Schmidt P. The 2012 hormone therapy position statement of The North American Menopause Society. Menopause. 2012;19(3):257–271.
3. https://www.medicalnewstoday.com/articles/155651.php - accessed 1/6/18.
4. Booth-LaForce C, Thurston RC, Taylor MR. A pilot study of a Hatha yoga treatment for menopausal symptoms. Maturitas. 2007;57:286–295.
5. Chattha R, Raghuram N, Venkatram P, Hongasandra NR. Treating the climacteric symptoms in Indian women with an integrated approach to yoga therapy: a randomized control study. Menopause. 2008;15:862–870.
6. Carson JW, Carson KM, Porter LS, Keefe FJ, Seewaldt VL. Yoga of Awareness program for menopausal symptoms in breast cancer survivors: results from a randomized trial. Support Care Cancer. 2009;17:1301–1309.
7. Afonso RF, Hachul H, Kozasa EH, et al. Yoga decreases insomnia in postmenopausal women: a randomized clinical trial. Menopause. 2012;19:186–193.
8. Reed SD, Guthrie KA, Newton KM, et al. Menopausal Quality of Life: A RCT of Yoga, Exercise and Omega-3 Supplements. American journal of obstetrics and gynecology. 2014;210(3):244.e1-244.e11. doi:10.1016/j.ajog.2013.11.016.
9. Jayabharathi B, Judie A. Complementary health approach to quality of life in menopausal women: a community-based interventional study. Clinical Interventions in Aging. 2014;9:1913-1921.
10. Vaze N, Joshi S. Yoga and menopausal transition. Indian Menopause Society. J Midlife Health. 2010;1:56–58.
11. Mastrangelo MA, Galantino ML, Chaloupka EC. Effects of yoga on quality of life and flexibility in perimenopausal and postmenopausal women. Med Sci Sports Exerc. 2005;37:s75.
12. Elavsky S, McAuley E. Physical activity and mental health outcomes during menopause: a randomized controlled trial. Annals of Behavioral Medicine. 2007;33(2):132–142.

13. Afonso RF, Hachul H, Kozasa EH, et al. Yoga decreases insomnia in postmenopausal women: a randomized clinical trial. Menopause. 2012;19:186–193.

14. Buchanan DT, Landis CA, Hohensee C, et al. Effects of Yoga and Aerobic Exercise on Actigraphic Sleep Parameters in Menopausal Women with Hot Flashes. Journal of Clinical Sleep Medicine: JCSM: Official Publication of the American Academy of Sleep Medicine. 2017;13(1):11-18. doi:10.5664/jcsm.6376.

15. Newton KM, Reed SD, Guthrie KA, et al. Efficacy of Yoga for Vasomotor Symptoms: A Randomized Controlled Trial. Menopause (New York, NY). 2014;21(4):339-346.

16. Avis NE, Legault C, Russell G, Weaver K, Danhauer SC. A Pilot Study of Integral Yoga for Menopausal Hot Flashes. Menopause (New York, NY). 2014;21(8):846-854.

17. Cramer H, Lauche R, Langhorst J, Dobos G. Effectiveness of Yoga for Menopausal Symptoms: A Systematic Review and Meta-Analysis of Randomized Controlled Trials. Evidence-based Complementary and Alternative Medicine: eCAM. 2012;2012:863905. doi:10.1155/2012/863905.

Menstrual Disorders

Menarche (the start of menstrual periods in women) in the West occurs around 14 years of age[1]. Normal menstruation (after the third year following menarche) is associated with an interval between periods in the range of 21–34 days, with a flow lasting from 3 to 7 days and a mean menstrual blood loss of 35 ml (range 5–80 ml)[2].

Menstrual disorders include: dysmenorrhea (painful cramps during menstruation), menorrhagia (excessive or prolonged bleeding during menstrual periods), amenorrhea (no menstruation by age 16 or no periods for at least 3 months while being regular before) and oligomenorrhea (periods occurring more than 35 days apart). Several systemic diseases may be associated with menstrual disorders and include, polycystic ovarian syndrome, Cushing's disease, thyroid dysfunction, adrenal tumors, prolactinomas, von Willebrand disease, and endometriosis[3]. Treatment is aimed at relieving pain in dysmenorrhea with the use of analgesics and NSAIDs. Heavy bleeding may be treated with oral contraceptives (especially Natazia) or LNG-IUS, an intrauterine device. Surgical interventions include endometrial ablation and rarely hysterectomy. Patients also use complementary and alternative medicine modalities, especially for peri-menstrual pain[4]. Yoga has also been tried as a therapeutic modality in menstrual disorders.

Yoga and Menstrual Disorders

Yoga nidra (yogic sleep) was tried in patients with menstrual disorders. One hundred and fifty patients were randomly divided into two groups – a control group of 75, and a yoga group of 75 (yoga nidra intervention, 35-minutes /day, five days in week). After six months, the yoga group demonstrated significant improvement in pain symptoms, gastrointestinal symptoms, cardiovascular symptoms, and urogenital symptoms, in comparison to control group[5].

In a study of premenstrual symptoms (menstrual pain was reported by 90.6% of the participants), sixty- four women were given yoga intervention. After 12 weeks, the participants reported decreased use of analgesics during menstruation and decreased effects of menstrual pain on work. They also noticed an improved functionality and decreased body pain. There was significantly decreased abdominal swelling, breast tenderness, abdominal cramps, and cold sweats[6].

In another study, fifty-eight students with premenstrual syndrome were divided into three groups: 20 in the yoga group (yoga practice 45 minutes daily, five days a week, for three months), 20 in the calcium group (500 mg, of calcium carbonate orally daily for three months) and18 in a control group. At the end of the study, the investigators reported a significant decrease in number and severity of premenstrual symptoms in the yoga (and calcium) group when compared to the control group[7].

Conclusion

Yoga may have a place in the adjunct treatment of menstrual disorders.

References

1. Wyshak G, Frisch RE. Evidence for a secular trend in age of menarche. N Engl J Med. 1982;306(17):1033–1035. doi: 10.1056/NEJM198204293061707.
2. ACOG Committee on Adolescent Health Care. Menstruation in girls and adolescents using the menstrual cycle as a vital sign. Obstet Gynecol. 2006;108(5):1323–1328. doi: 10.1097/00006250-200611000-00059.
3. Rigon F, De Sanctis V, Bernasconi S, et al. Menstrual pattern and menstrual disorders among adolescents: an update of the Italian data. Italian Journal of Pediatrics. 2012;38:38. doi:10.1186/1824-7288-38-38.
4. Fisher C, Adams J, Hickman L, Sibbritt D. The use of complementary and alternative medicine by 7427 Australian women with cyclic perimenstrual pain and discomfort: a cross-sectional study. BMC Complementary and Alternative Medicine. 2016;16:129. doi:10.1186/s12906-016-1119-8.
5. Rani K, Tiwari SC, Singh U, Agrawal GG, Srivastava N. Six-month trial of Yoga Nidra in menstrual disorder patients: Effects on somatoform symptoms. Industrial Psychiatry Journal. 2011;20(2):97-102. doi:10.4103/0972-6748.102489.
6. Premenstrual symptoms: Effect of Yoga Exercise on Premenstrual Symptoms among Female Employees in Taiwan. Su-Ying Tsai. Int J Environ Res Public Health. 2016 Jul; 13(7): 721. Published online 2016 Jul 16. doi: 10.3390/ijerph13070721.
7. Comparing the Effects of Yoga & Oral Calcium Administration in Alleviating Symptoms of Premenstrual Syndrome in Medical

Undergraduates. Mehta Bharati.J Caring Sci. 2016 Sep; 5(3): 179–185. Published online 2016 Sep 1. doi: 10.15171/jcs.2016.019.PMCID: PMC5045951.

Metabolic Syndrome

Metabolic syndrome is a cluster of metabolic abnormalities: impaired glucose metabolism, dyslipidemia, abdominal obesity, and elevated blood pressure[1]. It doubles the risk of mortality from cardiovascular diseases such as, coronary heart disease, stroke, and vascular dysfunction[2]. It results in a 5-fold increase in the risk of type 2 diabetes mellitus[3]. Patients with metabolic syndrome also have a higher all-cause mortality[4]. Diagnosis is made using one of several criteria advanced by professional associations[5]. According to the American Heart Association, metabolic syndrome is characterized by: waist circumference for males >40in, females>35in, fasting TG≥150mg/dL or treatment of this lipid abnormality, HDL<40mg/dL in males and <50mg/dL in females or treatment for this lipid abnormality, hypertension BP>130/85mm Hg or taking medication for hypertension and fasting glucose >100mg/dL or taking medicine for high glucose[6]. It is estimated that based on these criteria, almost 35% of US adults, and 50% of those older than 60 years old, have metabolic syndrome[7].

Treatment (with pharmacotherapy) is aimed at the major risk factors, namely elevated low-density lipoprotein cholesterol levels, hypertension, and diabetes[8]. Lifestyle changes, weight loss, prudent diet and adequate exercise also help, both in its prevention and in its treatment. Complementary and alternative medicine modalities have been used to treat this syndrome[9,10]. Several trials have also looked at the benefits of yoga practice in this syndrome[11-13].

Yoga and Metabolic Syndrome

A randomized case control study demonstrated that a 3-month yoga intervention in 101 middle aged adult patents induced significant improvements of several metabolic syndrome parameters. These included a reduction of waist circumference, systolic/diastolic blood pressure, fasting blood sugar level, HbA1c, serum triglyceride and an increase in the high-density lipoprotein-cholesterol from baseline to the end of the study period. A comparison to the control group was not given[14].

Another randomized controlled pilot study has further illustrated the feasibility and acceptability of yoga intervention in sedentary overweight adults with metabolic syndrome. The yoga group reported a significant improvement in energy level[15].

In a study of 283 adults, participants were randomized, and assigned to a control group of 137 and a yoga group of 146. The study was completed by 182 participants. After a year of yoga intervention, there was improvement in waist measurements and systolic blood pressure[16]. Another study also showed improvement in several metabolic parameters after a 12-week Hatha yoga intervention: 173 Chinese men and women aged 18 or above were assigned to two groups: yoga intervention group (n = 87) or a control group (n = 86). At the end of the study, yoga group participants achieved greater decline in waist circumference, fasting glucose, and triglycerides. Yoga training also improved general health perceptions, physical component scores, and social functioning domains scores of health-related qualities of life[17]. Another study looking at quality of life with yoga in metabolic syndrome patients also reported an improvement in these patients[18].

Paul-Labrador and colleagues reported beneficial effects of transcendental meditation using a two-group, parallel design in individuals with coronary heart disease and the metabolic syndrome. At the end of the study, the participants in the transcendental meditation group, when compared to a health education group, showed improvements in blood pressure, plasma glucose and insulin levels[19]. Anderson and Taylor reviewed three clinical trials addressing the use of mind-body therapies for management of the metabolic syndrome. Findings from the studies reviewed support the potential clinical effectiveness of mind-body practices in improving indices of the metabolic syndrome[20].

Other studies have demonstrated improvements with yoga, on stress[21], fasting blood sugar[22], and oxygen requirements during resting conditions with enhanced recovery after stress[23] in patients with the metabolic syndrome.

Conclusion

Yoga intervention improves several harmful parameters in patients with the metabolic syndrome. It also improves their quality of life.

References

1. Balkau B, Charles MA. Comment on the provisional report from the WHO consultation. European Group for the Study of Insulin Resistance (EGIR) Diabet Med. 1999;16:442–443.
2. Ford ES. The metabolic syndrome and mortality from cardiovascular disease and all-causes: findings from the National Health and Nutrition Examination Survey II Mortality Study. Atherosclerosis. 2004;173:309–14.
3. Alberti KGMM, Eckel RH, Grundy SM, et al. Harmonizing the metabolic syndrome: a joint interim statement of the international diabetes federation task force on epidemiology and prevention; National heart, lung, and blood institute; American heart association; World heart federation; International atherosclerosis society; And international association for the study of obesity. Circulation. 2009;120(16):1640–1645.
4. Wu SH, Liu Z, Ho SC. Metabolic syndrome and all-cause mortality: a meta-analysis of prospective cohort studies. Eur J Epidemiol. 2010 Jun;25(6):375-84. doi: 10.1007/s10654-010-9459-z. Epub 2010 Apr 28.
5. Srikanthan K, Feyh A, Visweshwar H, Shapiro JI, Sodhi K. Systematic Review of Metabolic Syndrome Biomarkers: A Panel for Early Detection, Management, and Risk Stratification in the West Virginian Population. International Journal of Medical Sciences. 2016;13(1):25-38. doi:10.7150/ijms.13800.
6. Scott M. Grundy, James I. Cleeman, Stephen R. Daniels, Karen A. Donato, Robert H. Eckel, Barry A. Franklin, David J. Gordon, Ronald M. Krauss, Peter J. Savage, Sidney C. Smith, John A. Spertus, Fernando Costa. Diagnosis and Management of the Metabolic Syndrome. An American Heart Association/National Heart, Lung, and Blood Institute Scientific Statement. Circulation. 2005;112:2735-2752.
7. Aguilar M, Bhuket T, Torres S, Liu B, Wong RJ. Prevalence of the metabolic syndrome in the United States, 2003-2012. Jama. 2015;313:1973–4.
8. Carrie Armstrong. AHA and NHLBI Review Diagnosis and Management of the Metabolic Syndrome Am Fam Physician. 2006 Sep 15;74(6):1039-1047.
9. Graf BL, Raskin I, Cefalu WT, Ribnicky DM. Plant-derived therapeutics for the treatment of metabolic syndrome. Current opinion in investigational drugs (London, England: 2000). 2010;11(10):1107-1115.
10. Jang S, Jang B-H, Ko Y, et al. Herbal Medicines for Treating Metabolic Syndrome: A Systematic Review of Randomized Controlled Trials.

Evidence-based Complementary and Alternative Medicine: eCAM. 2016;2016:5936402. doi:10.1155/2016/5936402.

11. Chaya M, Kurpad A, Nagendra H, Nagarathna R: The effect of long term combined yoga practice on the basal metabolic rate of healthy adults. BMC Complement Altern Med. 2006, 6 (1): 28-10.1186/1472-6882-6-28.

12. Chaya M, Nagendra H: Long-term effect of yogic practices on diurnal metabolic rates of healthy subjects. Int J Yoga. 2008, 1 (1): 27-10.4103/0973-6131.36761.

13. Swathi Gowda, Sriloy Mohanty, Apar Saoji, Raghuram Nagarathna. Integrated Yoga and Naturopathy module in management of Metabolic Syndrome: A case report. J Ayurveda Integr Med. 2017 Jan-Mar; 8(1): 45–48. Published online 2017 Mar 16. doi: 10.1016/j.jaim.2016.10.006.

14. Khatri D, Mathur KC, Gahlot S, Jain S, Agrawal RP. Effects of yoga and meditation on clinical and biochemical parameters of metabolic syndrome. Diabetes Res Clin Pract. 2007;78:e9–10. doi: 10.1016/j.diabres.2007.05.002.

15. SCohen BE, Chang AA, Grady D, Kanaya AM. Restorative yoga in adults with metabolic syndrome: a randomized, controlled pilot trial. Metab Syndr Relat Disord. 2008;6:223–9. doi: 10.1089/met.2008.0016.

16. Parco M Siu, Angus P Yu, Iris F Benzie, Jean Woo. Effects of 1-year yoga on cardiovascular risk factors in middle-aged and older adults with metabolic syndrome: a randomized trial. Diabetol Metab Syndr. 2015; 7: 40. Published online 2015 Apr 30. doi: 10.1186/s13098-015-0034-3.

17. Effects of a 12-Week Hatha Yoga Intervention on Metabolic Risk and Quality of Life in Hong Kong Chinese Adults with and without Metabolic SyndromeCaren Lau, Ruby Yu, Jean Woo.PLoS One. 2015; 10(6): e0130731.

18. Stephanie J. Sohl, Kenneth A. Wallston, Keiana Watkins, Gurjeet S. Birdee. Yoga for Risk Reduction of Metabolic Syndrome: Patient-Reported Outcomes from a Randomized Controlled Pilot Study. Evid Based Complement Alternat Med. 2016; 2016: 3094589.

19. Paul-Labrador M, Polk D, Dwyer JH, et al. Effects of a randomized controlled trial of transcendental meditation on components of the metabolic syndrome in subjects with coronary heart disease. Archives of Internal Medicine. 2006;166(11):1218–1224.

20. Anderson JG, Taylor AG. The Metabolic Syndrome and Mind-Body Therapies: A Systematic Review. Journal of Nutrition and Metabolism. 2011;2011:276419. doi:10.1155/2011/276419.

21. Corey SM, Epel E, Schembri M, et al. Effect of restorative yoga vs. stretching on diurnal cortisol dynamics and psychosocial outcomes in individuals with the metabolic syndrome: the PRYSMS randomized controlled trial. Psychoneuroendocrinology. 2014;49:260-271. doi:10.1016/j. psyneuen.2014.07.012.

22. Corey SM, Epel E, Schembri M, et al. Effect of restorative yoga vs. stretching on diurnal cortisol dynamics and psychosocial outcomes in individuals with the metabolic syndrome: the PRYSMS randomized

controlled trial. Psychoneuroendocrinology. 2014;49:260-271. doi:10.1016/j. psyneuen.2014.07.012.

23. Anupama Tyagi, Marc Cohen, John Reece, Shirley Telles. An explorative study of metabolic responses to mental stress and yoga practices in yoga practitioners, non-yoga practitioners and individuals with metabolic syndrome. BMC Complement Altern Med. 2014; 14: 445. Published online 2014 Nov 15. doi: 10.1186/1472-6882-14-445.

Migraine

Migraine is a common malady. It affects about 12-13 percent of the U.S. population (about 37 million). Of these, about 5 million sufferers experience at least one migraine attack per month. A migraine attack prevents 91 percent of the sufferers from going to work. It primarily affects people between the ages of 35 to 55 and is three times as common in women as men. Worldwide, it is the third most common disease and is in the top ten causes of disability[1].

Symptoms include moderate to severe pain, usually throbbing or pulsing, on one side of the head. This is accompanied by light and sound sensitivity and may result in nausea and vomiting (nausea is the most characteristic feature accompanying the headaches). Attacks are sometimes preceded by an aura. The attacks may be aggravated by physical activity and last from hours to 2-3 days. Because of the multi-sensory disturbance, the cause is attributed to an inherited dysfunction of sensory modulatory networks in the sub-cortical areas of the brain[2]. These patients also manifest chronic sympathetic dysfunction[3].

Many things can trigger a migraine. These include, anxiety, stress, lack of food or sleep, exposure to light and hormonal changes[4]. Migraine sufferers often have depression as a co-morbidity (seen in 30% of patients)[5]. Anxiety and panic attacks are also common in these patients[6]. Migraine is also linked to stress[7], and many other medical conditions like stroke, gastrointestinal disorders, and cardiovascular disease[8]. Migraine sufferers also experience poor quality of sleep[9]. Migraine with aura in women may also be a risk factor for cardio- and cerebro- vascular diseases[10]. Migraine patients have a poorer quality of life, when compared to the healthy population[11].

Treatment may be preventive or acute (abortive) or both[12]. First line treatment is usually nonprescription nonsteroidal anti-inflammatory drugs and combination analgesics containing acetaminophen, aspirin, and caffeine. For mild to moderate migraine, triptans are often prescribed. Severe attacks with significant nausea and vomiting may require intravenous antiemetics, with or without intravenous dihydroergotamine. Desamethasone is a good preventive agent and intranasal lidocaine may help acute migraine. Other drugs used include isometheptene-containing compounds and intranasal dihydroergotamine[13].

Treatment is often unsatisfactory and over 50% of these patients either self-medicate using non-prescription (over-the-counter) medication and do not seek medical help[14]. Complementary and alternative medicine modalities are often used by migraine sufferers[15].

Yoga and Migraine

Complimentary medicine, including yoga, has been beneficial in patients with migraine headaches[16,17].

John and associates performed a randomized controlled trial of seventy-two patients (migraine sufferers without aura) and assigned them to yoga therapy or self-care. After three months, the yoga group (compared to the self-care group) showed improvements in headache intensity, frequency, pain rating index, affective pain rating index, total pain rating index, and anxiety and depression scores. The yoga group also used fewer medications.

Kisan and associates studied the benefit of yoga in migraine patients. Sixty patients were randomly given either conventional care (n = 30) or yoga (5 days a week for 6 weeks) in addition to conventional care (n = 30). At the end of the study, the yoga group showed significant clinical improvement in headache frequency and intensity. The yoga group patients also manifested a reduction in the sympathetic tone and an enhancement in the vagal (parasympathetic) tone[18].

In another study, yoga was noted to improve endothelial function and have a beneficial effect on migraine. Migraine patients were enrolled and randomized into either a yoga exercise group (yoga plus medical treatment) or a control group (medical treatment alone). After 12 weeks, data was analyzed on 32 participants. Patients in the yoga group showed a significant improvement in vascular function, as elicited by a decrease in plasma levels of vascular cell adhesion molecule when compared with the control group[19].

Relaxation techniques, as often practiced during the corpse pose in yoga, may be helpful in migraine headache. The benefit of relaxation training in both migraine and tension type headache has been shown, with studies showing that on average, 43% to 55% of individuals experience 50% or greater reduction in headache frequency[20]. There were no yoga relaxation related migraine reduction studies on database searches.

Meditation, especially mindfulness based stress reduction (MBSR) has shown benefit in migraine patients. A randomized controlled trial with 19 episodic migraine patients, randomized to either MBSR (n = 10) or usual care (n = 9) for eight weeks revealed a beneficial effect on headache duration, disability, self-efficacy, and mindfulness, as secondary outcomes, in the former group[21].

Conclusion

Yoga may help prevent and/or relieve migraine headaches.

References

1. Steiner TJ et al. Migraine: the seventh disabler. The Journal of Headache and Pain 2013, 14:1.
2. Goadsby PJ et al. Neurobiology of migraine. Neuroscience 2009; 161(2): 327-41.
3. Peroutka SJ. Migraine: a chronic sympathetic nervous system disorder. Headache. 2004 Jan;44(1):53-64.
4. Kelman L. The triggers or precipitants of the acute migraine attack. Cephalalgia. 2007;27:394–402.
5. World Health Organization. Headache disorders. Fact sheet no.277, 2012.
6. Smitherman TA, Kolivas ED, Bailey JR. Panic disorder and migraine: comorbidity, mechanisms, and clinical implications. Headache. 2013;53:23–45.
7. Radat F. Stress and migraine. Revue neurologique. 2013;169:406–412.
8. Strine TW, Chapman DP, Balluz LS. Population-based US study of severe headaches in adults: psychological distress and comorbidities. Headache. 2006;46:223–232.
9. Lin Y-K, Lin G-Y, Lee J-T, et al. Associations Between Sleep Quality and Migraine Frequency: A Cross-Sectional Case-Control Study. Cuadrado. ML, ed. Medicine. 2016;95(17):e3554. doi:10.1097/MD.0000000000003554.

10. Kurth T, Gaziano JM, Cook NR, Logroscino G, Diener HC, Buring JE. Migraine and risk of cardiovascular disease in women. JAMA. 2006;296:283–91.

11. Dahlöf CG. Migraine patients experience poorer subjective well-being/quality of life even between attacks. Cephalalgia 1995;15(1):31-36.

12. Silberstein, S. D. (2012, December 05). Emerging Target-Based Paradigms to Prevent and Treat Migraine. Clinical Pharmacology and Therapeutics, 93(1):78-85. Retrieved April 17, 2017, from http://onlinelibrary.wiley.com/doi/10.1038/clpt.2012.198/abstract. Accessed 11/23/17.

13. Gilmore, B., & Michael, M. (2011, February 01). Treatment of acute migraine headache. American Academy of Family Physicians, 2011 Feb 1;83(3):271-280.

14. Headache Disorders – not respected, not resourced. All-Party Parliamentary Group on Primary Headache Disorders. 2010.

15. Crawford CC, Huynh MT, Kepple A, Jonas WB. Systematic assessment of the quality of research studies of conventional and alternative treatments of primary headache. Pain Physician. 2009;12:461–470.

16. Wells RE, Bertisch SM, Buettner C, Phillips RS, McCarthy EP. Complementary and alternative medicine use among adults with migraines/severe headaches. Headache. 2011 Jul-Aug;51(7):1087-97. doi: 10.1111/j.1526-4610.2011.01917.x. Epub 2011 Jun 7.

17. Millstine D, Chen CY, Bauer B. Complementary and integrative medicine in the management of headache. BMJ. 2017 May 16;357:j1805. doi: 10.1136/bmj.j1805.

18. Kisan R, Sujan M, Adoor M, et al. Effect of Yoga on migraine: A comprehensive study using clinical profile and cardiac autonomic functions. International Journal of Yoga. 2014;7(2):126-132. doi:10.4103/0973-6131.133891.

19. Naji-Esfahani H, Zamani M, Marandi SM, Shaygannejad V, Javanmard SH. Preventive Effects of a Three-month Yoga Intervention on Endothelial Function in Patients with Migraine. International Journal of Preventive Medicine. 2014;5(4):424-429.

20. Nicholson RA, Buse DC, Andrasik F, Lipton RB. Nonpharmacologic treatments for migraine and tension-type headache: how to choose and when to use. Curr Treat Options Neurol. 2011;13:28–40.

21. Wells RE, Burch R, Paulsen RH, Wayne PM, Houle TT, Loder E. Meditation for migraines: a pilot randomized controlled trial. Headache. 2014 Oct;54(9):1484-95. doi: 10.1111/head.12420. Epub 2014 Jul 18.

Multiple Sclerosis

Multiple sclerosis (MS) is an immune-mediated chronic inflammatory disease of the central nervous system[1]. It is estimated that 2.5 million people suffer from MS worldwide. It is more common in females[1]. It often leads to early disability in 20-25 years in more than 30% of the patients. Clinical manifestations include sensory disturbances, eye symptoms such as diplopia on lateral gaze and those associated with optic neuritis, spinal cord symptoms such as bladder and bowel dysfunction, cerebellar symptoms such as tremor and difficulties in coordination and balance, and cerebral symptoms such as cognitive dysfunction. They also suffer from fatigue, pain, depression and sleep disorders[2]. Their quality of life is usually poor[3]. Life expectancy may be reduced by 7-14 years[4].

Diagnostic testing includes MRI and evaluation of the cerebro-spinal fluid (CSF) examination via lumbar puncture (for oligoclonal bands and intrathecal immunoglobulin G (IgG) production). Evoked potentials and optical coherence tomography may also be used[5]. Treatment is directed at the immune dysfunction with immunomodulatory therapy. Therapy is also given to relieve or modify symptoms[6]. Drugs used include interferons, glatiramer acetate, fingolimod, mitoxantrone, natalizumab and others[7,8]. Vitamin D use has also been considered in these patients[9].

Complementary and alternative medicine is used by 33–65% of patients with multiple sclerosis[10,11]. Yoga has also been used in these patients for symptom relief[12], and other benefits[13].

Yoga and Multiple Sclerosis

Several studies have established the beneficial effects of yoga in patients with multiple sclerosis. Improvement has been reported in depression, pain, fatigue, lung capacity, strength and flexibility, stress, and quality of life[14,15]. Better bladder function has also been reported[16].

In a study of 69 patients with multiple sclerosis, Oken and associates found that in the 57 patients who completed the 6-

month study, patients in the exercise class (both Iyengar yoga and stationary bike) showed significant improvement in measures of fatigue when compared to a waiting-list control group[17].

Ahmadi and associates studied the effect of yoga in 31 MS patients. They were randomly assigned to one of three groups: treadmill training, yoga or control. Treadmill training and yoga practice (24 sessions, thrice weekly) for a period of eight weeks, while the control group followed their own routine treatment program. Objective measurements were made using the Berg Balance scores, time for 10-minute walk and distance covered during a two-minute walk, Fatigue Severity Scale (FSS), Beck Depression Inventory (BDI) and Beck Anxiety Inventor (BAI) were used for the evaluation. At the end of the study, both exercise groups (yoga and treadmill) showed significant improvements in the balance score, walking endurance, FFS score, BDI score and BAI score. Anxiety was much improved in the yoga group compared to the treadmill training group. Quality of life was also better in the yoga group[18].

In a study of 20 subjects, 25-50 years of age, with relapsing-remitting or progressive MS, evaluation after 10 weeks showed some improvement in selective attention performance in the yoga group. No benefit was noted on mood or fatigue[19].

Yoga may also relieve pain and depression and improve the quality of life in patients with multiple sclerosis[20,21].

Cramer and group performed a meta-analysis of seven randomized controlled trials (yoga and multiple sclerosis) involving a total of 670 patients. They found that yoga practice was associated with a beneficial effect on symptoms of fatigue, quality of life, muscle function, or cognitive function. No benefits were noted compared to exercise. They recommended the use of yoga in patients with multiple sclerosis, if regular exercise was not tolerated. There were no serious adverse events reported[22].

Gunner and associates in a study involving eight MS patients, found that after 12 weeks of a bi-weekly yoga program, participants showed improvement in fatigue, balance and spatiotemporal gait parameters. The researchers used the Fatigue

Severity Scale and Berg Balance Scale to assess fatigue and balance[23].

Multiple sclerosis patients do not tolerate hot temperatures well and they should avoid Bikram yoga[24].

Conclusion

Yoga like regular exercise is efficacious in reducing fatigue and improving the quality of life in patients with multiple sclerosis. MS patients may prefer yoga over regular exercise.

References

1. Compston A, Coles A. Multiple sclerosis. Lancet. 2008;372:1502–1517. doi: 10.1016/S0140-6736(08)61620-7.
2. Zwibel HL. Contribution of impaired mobility and general symptoms to the burden of multiple sclerosis. Adv Ther 2009;26:n1043–1057.
3. Orme M, Kerrigan J, Tyas D, Russell N, Nixon R. The effect of disease, functional status, and relapses on the utility of people with multiple sclerosis in the UK. Value Health. 2007;10:54–60.
4. Kingwell E, van der Kop M, Zhao Y, Shirani A, Zhu F, Oger J, Tremlett H. Relative mortality and survival in multiple sclerosis: findings from British Columbia, Canada.J Neurol Neurosurg Psychiatry. 2012 Jan; 83(1):61-6.
5. Polman CH, Reingold SC, Banwell B, Clanet M, Cohen JA, Filippi M, Fujihara K, Havrdova E, Hutchinson M, Kappos L, Lublin FD, Montalban X, O'Connor P, Sandberg-Wollheim M, Thompson AJ, Waubant E, Weinshenker B, Wolinsky JS. Diagnostic criteria for multiple sclerosis: 2010 revisions to the McDonald criteria. Ann Neurol. 2011;69:292–302. doi: 10.1002/ana.22366.
6. Vosoughi R, Freedman MS. Therapy of MS. Clin Neurol Neurosurg. 2010 Jun;112(5):365-85. doi: 10.1016/j.clineuro.2010.03.010. Epub 2010 Apr 1.
7. Clerico M, Rivoiro C, Contessa G, Viglietti D, Durelli L. The therapy of multiple sclerosis with immune-modulating or immunosuppressive drug. A critical evaluation based upon evidence based parameters and published systematic reviews. Clin Neurol Neurosurg. 2008 Nov;110(9):878-85. doi: 10.1016/j.clineuro.2007.10.020. Epub 2008 Mar 4.
8. Buck D, Hemmer B. Treatment of multiple sclerosis: current concepts and future perspectives. J Neurol. 2011;258:1747–1762. doi: 10.1007/s00415-011-6101-2.
9. Dörr J, Döring A, Paul F. Can we prevent or treat multiple sclerosis by individualised vitamin D supply? The EPMA Journal. 2013;4(1):4. doi:10.1186/1878-5085-4-4.

10. Winterholler M, Erbguth F, Neundorfer B. The use of alternative medicine by multiple sclerosis patients–patient characteristics and patterns of use. Fortschr Neurol Psychiatr. 1997;65:555–561.
11. Shinto L, Yadav V, Morris C, Lapidus JA, Senders A, Bourdette D. Demographic and health-related factors associated with complementary and alternative medicine (CAM) use in multiple sclerosis. Mult Scler. 2006;12:94–100.
12. Frank R, Larimore J. Yoga as a method of symptom management in multiple sclerosis. Frontiers in Neuroscience. 2015;9:133. doi:10.3389/fnins.2015.00133.
13. Mishra SK, Singh P, Bunch S, Zhang R. The therapeutic value of yoga in neurological disorders. Ann Indian Acad Neurol 2012;15:247–254.
14. Senders A, Wahbeh H, Spain R, Shinto L. Mind-body medicine for multiple sclerosis: a systematic review. Autoimmune Dis 2012;2012:567324.
15. Rogers KA, MacDonald M. Therapeutic Yoga: Symptom Management for Multiple Sclerosis. Journal of Alternative and Complementary Medicine. 2015;21(11):655-659. doi:10.1089/acm.2015.0015.
16. Patil NJ, Nagaratna R, Garner C, et al. Effect of integrated yoga on neurogenic bladder dysfunction in patients with multiple sclerosis: a prospective observational case series. Complement Ther Med 2012;20:424–430.
17. Oken BS, Kishiyama S, Zajdel D, Bourdette D, Carlsen J, et al. (2004) Randomized controlled trial of yoga and exercise in multiple sclerosis. Neurology 62: 2058–2064.
18. Ahmadi A, Nikbakh M, Arastoo A, Habibi AH (2010) The Effects of a yoga intervention on balance, speed and endurance of walking, fatigue and quality of life in people with multiple sclerosis. J Hum Kinet 23: 71–78.
19. Velikonja O, Curic K, Ozura A, Jazbec SS (2010) Influence of sports climbing and yoga on spasticity, cognitive function, mood and fatigue in patients with multiple sclerosis. Clin Neurol Neurosurg 112: 597–601.
20. Rahnama N, Namazizadeh M, Etemadifar M, Bambaeichi E, Arbabzadeh S, et al. (2011) Effects of yoga on depression in women with multiple sclerosis. Journal of Isfahan Medical School 29: 483–490.
21. Doulatabad SN, Nooreyan K, Doulatabad AN, Noubandegani ZM (2012) The effects of pranayama, hatha and raja yoga on physical pain and the quality of life of women with multiple sclerosis. Afr J Tradit Complement Altern Med 10: 49–52.
22. Cramer H, Lauche R, Azizi H, Dobos G, Langhorst J. Yoga for Multiple Sclerosis: A Systematic Review and Meta-Analysis. Manzoli L, ed. PLoS ONE. 2014;9(11):e112414. doi:10.1371/journal.pone.0112414.

23. Guner S, Inanici F. Yoga therapy and ambulatory multiple sclerosis assessment of gait analysis parameters, fatigue, and balance. J Body Move Ther 2015;19:72–81.
24. Guthrie TC, Nelson DA. Influence of temperature changes on multiple sclerosis: critical review of mechanisms and research potential. J Neurol Sci. 1995;129:1–8.

Obesity

Obesity is a global epidemic[1]. The Centers for Disease Control and Prevention defines obesity as a body mass index of 30 or greater[2]. It is estimated that over 2.1 billion people – nearly 30% of the world's population are either obese or overweight and these numbers are on the increase[3]. The reasons are numerous[4], and include genetic, metabolic, behavioral, and environmental factors[5]. Obesity transmits a significant disease burden on the human population – predominantly chronic diseases[6], and especially cardiovasculars[7,8]. Efforts to reduce weight are usually futile, despite medications[9]. Bariatric surgery is an effective option in these patients but is associated with potentially severe complications[10].

Lifestyle changes aimed at weight reduction through physical activity, proper diet, breathing exercises and stress relaxation appear to provide better results at weight reduction and the associated metabolic complications[11]. Practice of yoga is one such lifestyle change.

Yoga and Obesity

Yoga is commonly used as a complementary modality for weight control[12], decreasing body mass index (BMI)[13] and for improving body composition[14,15]. Several studies have also shown a reduction in central obesity with yoga practice, with or without weight loss[16].

In a coronary artery disease study involving 42 men with angiographically proven coronary artery disease, yoga intervention (along with diet control, control of risk factors and moderate aerobic exercise) for a duration of one year in 21 men in the yoga group resulted in a decrease in body weight, when compared to the 21 men in the control group[17].

Yoga is effective in reducing the amount of weight gain. In a trial involving 15,550 adults, aged 53 to 57 years, participants were recruited to the Vitamin and Lifestyle cohort study. (2000 and 2002). The researchers found that both normal weight and overweight individuals had attenuated weight gain with yoga practice. Four or more years of yoga practice was associated with a 3.1-lb lower weight gain among normal weight participants and an 18.5-lb lower weight gain among overweight participants[18].

A review of data from 20 personal journals of 25 women with obesity, revealed that yoga was responsible for a positive shift in eating habits in these women, with an overall reduction in the quantity of food they consumed, decreased eating speed, and an improvement in food choices[19].

In a study[20] involving sixteen healthy postmenopausal obese women (8 yoga group and 8 control group), yoga exercise for 16 weeks was associated with a significant decrease in body weight, percentage of body fat, lean body mass, body mass index, waist circumference, and visceral fat area.

A 12-week yoga program in 40 obese women also demonstrated a reduction in central obesity, when compared to 20 obese controls. The yoga group achieved a reduction in the waist-hip ratio, body weight, BMI, and percentage of body fat and increased the percentage of body muscle[21].

In a study of obese breast cancer survivors[22], researchers recorded a decrease in waist circumference measurements with yoga practice.

In a 5-day residential Kripalu yoga study published in 2012, thirty-seven overweight/obese program participants (age 32-65, BMI<25) were evaluated for several parameters. One of them was body weight, which was monitored at baseline and 1 year after program completion. The researchers noted a significant self-reported weight loss at one year, in 19 of the respondents[23].

Twenty obese boys (body mass index greater than the 95th percentile) were studied for the effect of yoga on their body composition. They were randomly assigned to a yoga (n=10) and a control group (n=10). The former group underwent an 8-week of yoga-asana training. After yoga training, the yoga group were noted to have significantly decreased body weight, BMI, fat mass, and body fat percentage. They also significantly increased their fat-free mass and basal metabolic rate when compared to the baseline values[24].

A study of 4307 randomly selected individuals from 15 US Iyengar yoga studios, 53.7 % of the 1087 individuals who responded (1045 (24.3%) surveys completed), indicated that they had lost weight with yoga practice[25]. The greater the frequency of practice, the better the weight loss[26].

Mindfulness meditation is also effective in helping weight control, when used as a compliment to traditional weight loss programs, as was seen in 13 of the 19 studies reviewed[27]. In a narrative review, based on scientific published data, researchers concluded that yoga is beneficial in reducing weight[28].

Conclusion

Yoga appears to be an appropriate and potentially successful intervention for weight maintenance, prevention of obesity, and risk reduction for diseases in which obesity plays a significant causal role.

References

1. Caballero B. The global epidemic of obesity: an overview. Epidemiol Rev. 2007; 29:1–5.
2. CDC. Vital signs: state-specific obesity prevalence among adults— United States, 2009. Morbidity and Mortality Weekly Report. 2010;59:1–5.
3. Marie Ng, Tom Fleming, BS, Margaret Robinson et al. Global, regional, and national prevalence of overweight and obesity in children and adults during 1980–2013: a systematic analysis for the Global Burden of Disease Study 2013. Lancet, 2014, Volume 384, No. 9945, p766–781.
4. McAllister EJ, Dhurandhar NV, Keith SW, et al. Ten Putative Contributors to the Obesity Epidemic. Crit Rev Food Sci Nutr. 2009 Nov; 49(10): 868–913.
5. Wang Y, McPherson K, Marsh T, et al. Health and economic burden of the projected obesity trends in the USA and the UK. Lancet. 2011; 378:815–825.
6. Must A, Spadano J, Coakley EH, Field AE, et al. The disease burden associated with overweight and obesity. J Am Med Assoc. 1999; 282:1523.
7. Bray GA. Medical consequences of obesity. J Clin Endocrinol Metab. 2004; 89:2583–9.
8. Nakamura K, Fuster JJ, Kenneth Walsh K. Adipokines: A link between obesity and cardiovascular disease. J Cardiol. 2014 Apr; 63(4): 250–259.

9. Lewis K, Gudzune KA. Overcoming challenges to obesity counseling: suggestions for the primary care provider. Journal of Clinical Outcomes Management. 2014;21(3):123–133.

10. Arterburn D. E., Courcoulas A. P. Bariatric surgery for obesity and metabolic conditions in adults. The British Medical Journal. 2014;349 doi: 10.1136/bmj.g3961.g3961.

11. Goran MI, Alderete TL. Targeting adipose tissue inflammation to treat the underlying basis of the metabolic complications of obesity. Nestle Nutr Inst Workshop Ser. 2012; 73:49–60.

12. Sharpe PA, Blanck HM, Williams JE, Ainsworth BE, Conway JM. Use of complementary and alternative medicine for weight control in the United States. J Altern Complement Med. 2007;13:217–22.

13. Moliver N, Mika E, Chartrand M, Burrus S, Haussmann R, Khalsa S. Increased Hatha yoga experience predicts lower body mass index and reduced medication use in women over 45 years. International Journal of Yoga. 2011;4(2):77-86. doi:10.4103/0973-6131.85490.

14. Bera TK, Rajapurkar MV. Body composition, cardiovascular endurance and anaerobic power of yogic practitioner. Indian J Physiol Pharmacol. 1993; 37:225–8.

15. Dhananjay V. Arankalle, Madan S. Kumar. Effect of yoga techniques practice in obese adults. SENSE, 2013, Vol. 3 (3), 22-29.

16. Siu PM, Yu AP, Benzie IF, Woo J. Effects of 1-year yoga on cardiovascular risk factors in middle-aged and older adults with metabolic syndrome: a randomized trial. Diabetology & Metabolic Syndrome. 2015;7:40. doi:10.1186/s13098-015-0034-3.

17. Manchanda SC, Narang R, Reddy KS, Sachdeva U, Prabhakaran D, Dharmanand S, et al. Retardation of coronary atherosclerosis with yoga lifestyle intervention. J Assoc Physicians India. 2000;48:687–94.

18. Kristal AR, Littman AJ, Benitez D, White E. Yoga practice is associated with attenuated weight gain in healthy, middle-aged men and women. Altern Ther Health Med. 2005;11:28–33.

19. McIver S., McGartland M., O'Halloran P. 'Overeating is not about the food': women describe their experience of a yoga treatment program for binge eating. Qualitative Health Research. 2009;19(9):1234–1245. doi: 10.1177/1049732309343954.

20. Lee JA, Kim JW, Kim DY. Effects of yoga exercise on serum adiponectin and metabolic syndrome factors in obese postmenopausal women. Menopause. 2012;19:296–301.

21. Cramer H, Sushila Thoms M, Anheyer D, Lauche R, Dobos G. Yoga in Women With Abdominal Obesity— a Randomized Controlled Trial. Deutsches Ärzteblatt International. 2016;113(39):645-652.

22. Littman AJ, Bertram LC, Ceballos R, Ulrich CM, Ramaprasad J, McGregor B, et al. Randomized controlled pilot trial of yoga in overweight and obese breast cancer survivors: effects on quality of life and anthropometric measures. Support Care Cancer. 2012;20:267–77.

23. Braun TD, Park CL, Conboy LA. Psychological well-being, health behaviors, and weight loss among participants in a residential, Kripalu yoga-based weight loss program. Int J Yoga Therap. 2012;22:9–22.

24. Seo DY, Lee S, Figueroa A, Kim HK, Baek YH, Kwak YS, et al. Yoga training improves metabolic parameters in obese boys. Korean J Physiol Pharmacol. 2012;16:175–80.
25. Ross A., Friedmann E., Bevans M., Thomas S. National survey of yoga practitioners: mental and physical health benefits. Complementary Therapies in Medicine. 2013;21(4):313–323. doi: 10.1016/j.ctim.2013.04.001.
26. Ross A., Friedmann E., Bevans M., Thomas S. Frequency of yoga practice predicts health: results of a national survey of yoga practitioners. Evidence-based Complementary and Alternative Medicine. 2012;2012:10. doi: 10.1155/2012/983258.983258.
27. Olson K. L., Emery C. F. Mindfulness and weight loss: a systematic review. Psychosomatic Medicine. 2015;77(1):59–67.
28. Rioux JG, Ritenbaugh C. Narrative review of yoga intervention clinical trials including weight-related outcomes. Altern Ther Health Med. 2013 May-Jun;19(3):32-46.

Obsessive Compulsive Disorder

Obsessive compulsive disorder (OCD) is a common psychiatric condition. It is estimated that approximately 3.3 million people have OCD in the USA. It affects 0.3 to 1% of the pediatric population and 2% of the adult population[1]. It is associated with increased mortality and can have a substantial impact on quality of life for both patients and family members or caregivers[2].Obsessive-compulsive disorder (OCD) is a debilitating condition that afflicts approximately 1% to 3% of the world population and is the tenth leading cause of disability worldwide[3]. It is a high burden disease, and depression is common co-morbidity[4,5]. Other co-morbidities include anxiety, bipolar disorders, attention deficit hyperactivity disorder, eating disorders, autism spectrum disorder and tic disorders[6-8]. Most patients and caregivers experience a poor quality of life[9]. Patients with OCD also have a decreased life expectancy[10].

Patients with OCD experience the presence of recurrent, unwanted, and intrusive thoughts and/or manifest repetitive behaviors or rituals intended to relieve the fear, anxiety, and/or distress associated with their obsessions[11], resulting in significant distress and impairment in social, academic, and/or family functioning.

The primary treatments are selective serotonin reuptake inhibitors[12] and behavioral therapy[13,14]. OCD is difficult to treat. Approximately 30% to 40% of patients continue to have disabling OCD symptoms, despite therapy[15]. Yoga has been tried in these patients[16].

Yoga and OCD

In a study of eight patients with OCD, researchers prescribed one year of yogic breathing. Five patients completed the study. There was a significant improvement in these five at the end of the study, with three patients stopping medications and the other two reducing them[17].

Another trial measured the benefits of Kundilini yoga in patients with OCD. Twenty-two patients were randomly assigned to two groups. Group 1 (12 patients) employed a kundalini yoga meditation protocol and Group 2 (10 patients) employed the Relaxation Response plus Mindfulness Meditation technique. Seven patients completed the study in each group. The researchers used Yale-Brown Obsessive Compulsive Scale, Symptoms Checklist-90-Revised Obsessive Compulsive and Global Severity Index scale, Profile of Moods scale, Perceived Stress Scale, and Purpose in Life tests to evaluate these patients at baseline, 3 months, and 15 months. Groups were merged after 3 months. Patients under yoga therapy showed marked improvements, both before merging the groups, and after an additional one year, as part of the combined group[18].

Conclusion

Preliminary results show that yoga may allow patients with OCD feel better and help them reduce their medications.

References

1. http://understanding_ocd.tripod.com/ocd_facts_statistics.html - accessed 10/15/17.
2. Veale D, Roberts A. Obsessive-compulsive disorder. BMJ. 2014;348:g2183.; Fontenelle LF, Mendlowicz MV, Versiani M. The descriptive epidemiology of obsessive-compulsive disorder. Prog Neuropsychopharmacol Biol Psychiatry. 2006;30:327–337.
3. Sasson Y, Zohar J, Chopra M, Lustig M, Iancu I, Hendler T. Epidemiology of obsessive-compulsive disorder: a world view. J Clin Psychiatry. 1997;58 Suppl 12:7-10.
4. Hong JP, Samuels J, Bienvenu OJ, Cannistraro P, Grados M, Riddle MA, et al. Clinical correlates of recurrent major depression in obsessive–compulsive disorder. Depression and Anxiety. 2004;20:86–91. doi: 10.1002/da.20024.
5. Brown HM, Lester KJ, Jassi A, Heyman I, Krebs G. Paediatric Obsessive-Compulsive Disorder and Depressive Symptoms: Clinical Correlates and CBT Treatment Outcomes. Journal of Abnormal Child Psychology. 2015;43(5):933-942. doi:10.1007/s10802-014-9943-0.
6. Levy HC, McLean CP, Yadin E, Foa EB. Characteristics of individuals seeking treatment for obsessive-compulsive disorder. Behav Ther. 2013;44(3):408–416.
7. Lochner C, Fineberg NA, Zohar J, et al. Comorbidity in obsessive-compulsive disorder (OCD): a report from the International College of Obsessive-Compulsive Spectrum Disorders (ICOCS) Compr Psychiatry. 2014;55(7):1513–1519.

8. Hollander E, Stein DJ, Kwon JH, et al. Psychosocial functions and economic costs of obsessive-compulsive disorder. CNS Spectrums. 1997;2(10):16–25. doi: 10.1017/S1092852900011068.

9. Macy AS, Theo JN, Kaufmann SC. Quality of life in obsessive compulsive disorder. CNS Spectr. 2013;18:21–33.

10. Meier SM, Mattheisen M, Mors O, Schendel DE, Mortensen PB, Plessen KJ. Mortality among persons with obsessive-compulsive disorder in Denmark. JAMA Psychiatry. 2016;73:268–274.

11. APA. Diagnostic and Statistical Manual of Mental Disorders: DSM−5. Washington, DC: American Psychiatric Association; 2013.

12. Soomro GM, Altman D, Rajagopal S, Oakley-Browne M. Selective serotonin re-uptake inhibitors (SSRIs) versus placebo for obsessive compulsive disorder (OCD) Cochrane Database Syst Rev. 2008;1 CD001765.

13. Gava I, Barbui C, Aguglia E. Psychological treatments versus treatment as usual for obsessive compulsive disorder (OCD) Cochrane Database Sys Rev. 2007;2 CD005333.

14. Belotto-Silva C, Diniz JB, Malavazzi DM. Group cognitive-behavioral therapy versus selective serotonin reuptake inhibitors for obsessive-compulsive disorder: a practical clinical trial. J Anxiety Disord. 2012;26:25–31.

15. National Institute for Health and Care Excellence. Obsessive-compulsive disorder: core interventions in the treatment of obsessive-compulsive disorder and body dysmorphic disorder. National Institute for Health and Care Excellence; London: 2005.

16. da Silva TL, Ravindran LN, Ravindran AV. Yoga in the treatment of mood and anxiety disorders: A review. BMC Psychiatry. 2014; 14(Suppl 1): S1. Published online 2014 Jul 2. doi: 10.1186/1471-244X-14-S1-S1.

17. Shannahoff-Khalsa DS, Beckett LR. Clinical case report: efficacy of yogic techniques in the treatment of obsessive compulsive disorders. Int J Neurosci. 1996 Mar;85(1-2):1-17.

18. Shannahoff-Khalsa DS, Ray LE, Levine S, Gallen CC, Schwartz BJ, Sidorowich JJ. Randomized controlled trial of yogic meditation techniques for patients with obsessive-compulsive disorder. CNS Spectr. 1999 Dec;4(12):34-47.

Osteoarthritis

Arthritis affects almost 50 million Americans[1]. It is the nation's most common cause of disability[2]. Osteoarthritis (OA) is the most common form of arthritis, and is progressive and chronic in nature[3]. Worldwide, osteoarthritis is the most common joint disorder. In western countries, radiographic evidence of this disease is present in most persons by 65 years of age and in about 80 percent of persons more than 75 years of age[4]. It usually affects the spine, hands, hips and knees, while avoiding the wrists, elbows or shoulders[5]. It is a major cause of pain, disability, and reduced quality of life[6].

Symptoms include joint pain, morning stiffness lasting less than 30 minutes, joint instability or buckling, and loss of function. Physical examination may reveal bony enlargement at affected joints, limitation of range of motion, pain and crepitus on motion and joint malalignment or deformity[7].

The American College of Rheumatology has developed diagnostic criteria for osteoarthritis at various sites, including the hip[8], the knee[9] and the hand[5]. X-rays of the affected joint may show loss of joint space and the presence of new bone formation or osteophytes. Pharmacologic treatment includes drugs such as simple analgesics like tylenol[10], Opioid-containing analgesics, including codeine and propoxyphene, nonsteroidal anti-inflammatory drugs[11] and local analgesics like capsaicin cream. Intra-articular injections with corticosteroids or hyaluronic acid–like products (Hyalgan, Synvisc) may be required. Finally, surgical intervention may be needed[12]. Yoga has also shown promise in the adjunct treatment of osteoarthritis[13].

Yoga and Osteoarthritis

Yoga can be effective in reducing the pain and disability in osteoarthritis[14-16].

Haaz and associate reviewed eleven studies published from 1980 to 2010 on the role of yoga in arthritis (both osteoarthritis and rheumatoid arthritis). They found that yoga was effective in reducing disease symptoms (tender/swollen joints, pain) and disability. Patients also experienced improved self-efficacy and better mental health[17].

In a prospective, randomized, active controlled trial, 250 patients (ages 50-80 years) with OA of the knees were randomized into a hath yoga group and a control group (therapeutic exercises). Both groups underwent supervised intervention for 40 minutes per day, for 3 months. The yoga group demonstrated improvements in walking pain, range of knee flexion, walking time, tenderness, swelling, crepitus, and knee disability[18]. Another study also reported yoga related improvement in OA symptoms in older women (average age 72 years) with knee osteoarthritis[19].

In a study evaluating the efficacy of yoga on arthritis in sedentary people, researchers randomly assigned 75 adults aged 18+ with rheumatoid arthritis or knee osteoarthritis to 8 weeks of yoga (two 60 min classes and 1 home practice/week) or a waitlist. At the end of the study, yoga participants showed significant improvements in mean Physical Component Summary, flexibility, 6-minute walk, all psychological and most health-related quality of life domains. The authors also reported that most of these improvements were still evident 9 months later[20].

Pain is a prominent symptom in osteoarthritis. In a review of 9 articles (6 studies), with 372 subjects suffering from knee osteo-arthritis, Kan and co-researchers found yoga to be effective in relieving pain in these individuals. Most study patients followed a yoga protocol of 40~90 minutes/session, lasting for at least 8 weeks. Mobility was also improved in these patients[21].

Most of these studies have looked at the effects of yoga in patients with knee osteo-arthritis. The role of yoga in spinal degenerative arthritis is discussed in the chapter on back pain.

Conclusion

Yoga is effective in reducing the symptoms of osteoarthritis, increasing activity in patients and improving their quality of life.

References

1. Cheng YJ, Hootman JM, Murphy LB, Langmaid GA, Helmick CG. Prevalence of doctor-diagnosed arthritis and arthritis-attributable activity

limitation — United States, 2007–2009. Morb Mortal Wkly Rep. 2010;59(39):1261–1265.

2. Furner SE, Hootman JM, Helmick CG, Bolen J, Zack MM. Health-related quality of life of U.S. Adults with arthritis: analysis of data from the behavioral risk factor surveillance system, 2005, and 2007. Arthritis Care Res. 2003;2011:788–799.

3. Bijlsma JW, Berenbaum F, Lafeber FP. Osteoarthritis: an update with relevance for clinical practice. Lancet. 2011;377:2115–26.

4. Lawrence RC, Hochberg MC, Kelsey JL, McDuffie FC, Medsger TA Jr, Felts WR, et al. Estimates of the prevalence of selected arthritic and musculoskeletal diseases in the United States. J Rheumatol. 1989;16:427–41.

5. Altman R, Alarcon G, Appelrouth D, Bloch D, Borenstein D, Brandt K, et al. The American College of Rheumatology criteria for the classification and reporting of osteoarthritis of the hand. Arthritis Rheum. 1990;33(11):1601–1610. Epub 1990/11/01.

6. Arden N, Nevitt MC. Osteoarthritis: epidemiology. Best Pract Res Clin Rheumatol. 2006;20:3–25.

7. Nisha JM, Nancy EL. Osteoarthritis: Current Concepts in Diagnosis and Management. Am Fam Physician. 2000 Mar 15;61(6):1795-1804.

8. Altman R, Alarcon G, Appelrouth D, Bloch D, Borenstein D, Brandt K, et al. The American College of Rheumatology criteria for the classification and reporting of osteoarthritis of the hip. Arthritis Rheum. 1991;34:505–14.

9. Altman R, Asch E, Bloch D, Bole D, Borenstein K, Brandt K, et al. Development of criteria for the classification and reporting of osteoarthritis. Classification of osteoarthritis of the knee. Arthritis Rheum. 1986;29:1039–49.

10. Amadio P, Cummings DM. Evaluation of acetaminophen in the management of osteoarthritis of the knee. Curr Ther Res. 1983;34:59–66.

11. Furst DE. Are there differences among nonsteroidal antiinflammatory drugs? Comparing acetylated salicylates, nonacetylated salicylates, and nonacetylated nonsteroidal antiinflammatory drugs. Arthritis Rheum. 1994;37:1–9.

12. Buckwalter JA, Lohmander S. Operative treatment of osteoarthritis. Current practice and future development. J Bone Joint Surg [Am]. 1994;76:1405–18.

13. Sharma M. Yoga as an alternative and complementary approach for arthritis: A systematic review. Journal of Evidence-Based Complementary & Alternative Medicine. 2014;19:51–8.

14. Garfinkel MS, Schumacher HR, Jr, Husain A, Levy M, Reshetar RA. Evaluation of a yoga based regimen for treatment of osteoarthritis of the hands. The Journal of Rheumatology. 1994;21(12):2341–2343.

15. Kolasinski SL, Garfinkel M, Tsai AG. Iyengar Yoga for treating symptoms of osteoarthritis of the knees: a pilot study. J Alternative Compl Med. 2005;11:689–693. doi: 10.1089/acm.2005.11.689.

16. Bukowski EL, Conway A, Glentz LA, Kurland K, Galantino ML. The effect of Iyengar Yoga and strengthening exercises for people living with osteoarthritis of the knee: a case series. Int Q Community Health Educ. 2006;26:287–305.

17. Haaz S, Bartlett SJ. Yoga for arthritis: A scoping review. Rheum Dis Clin North Am. 2011;37:33–46.

18. Ebnezar J, Nagarathna R, Yogitha B, Nagendra HR. Effects of an integrated approach of hatha yoga therapy on functional disability, pain, and flexibility in osteoarthritis of the knee joint: a randomized controlled study. J Altern Complement Med. 2012;18(5):463–472. doi: 10.1089/acm.2010.0320. doi:10.1089/acm.2010.0320.

19. Cheung C, Wyman JF, Resnick B, Savik K. Yoga for managing knee osteoarthritis in older women: a pilot randomized controlled trial. BMC Complementary and Alternative Medicine. 2014;14:160. doi:10.1186/1472-6882-14-160.

20. Moonaz S, Bingham CO, Wissow L, Bartlett SJ. Yoga in sedentary adults with arthritis: effcts of a randomized controlled pragmatic trial. The Journal of rheumatology. 2015;42(7):1194-1202. doi:10.3899/jrheum.141129.

21. Kan L, Zhang J, Yang Y, Wang P. The Effects of Yoga on Pain, Mobility, and Quality of Life in Patients with Knee Osteoarthritis: A Systematic Review. Evidence-based Complementary and Alternative Medicine: eCAM. 2016;2016:6016532. doi:10.1155/2016/6016532.

Osteoporosis

Osteoporosis is a chronic and progressive disease characterized by low bone mass, microarchitecture deterioration of bone tissue, and bone fragility[1]. It is the most common bone disease in humans[2]. It is estimated that about 10 million Americans suffer from osteoporosis. Increasing age is a risk factor for this disease[3]. Patients with osteoporosis are at increased risk of osteoporotic fractures[4]. This results in an increased risk of disability and nursing home placement[5]. There is associated depression and loss of self-esteem in these patients[6]. Mortality also goes up, especially after hip fractures[7].

According to the World Health Organization[8] osteoporosis and osteopenia in postmenopausal women and men older than 50 years can be diagnosed by the following bone mass density (BMD) figures derived from DEXA (dual energy x-ray absorptiometry) measurements.

Normal: Spinal or hip BMD within 1.0 standard deviation (SD) below the young adult female reference mean (T-score ≥ −1.0)

Low bone mass (osteopenia): Spinal or hip BMD between 1.0 and 2.5 SDs below the young adult female reference mean (T-score < −1.0 and > −2.5)

Osteoporosis: Spinal or hip BMD ≥ 2.5 SDs below the young adult female reference mean (T-score ≤ −2.5)

Severe/established osteoporosis: BMD ≥ 2.5 SDs below the young adult female reference mean and the presence of one or more fragility fractures.

Pharmacologic treatment includes bisphosphonates, raloxifene, teriparatide, and denosumab[9]. Non-pharmacologic treatments are mainly directed towards fall prevention[10]. These include, alcohol moderation (less than 4 drinks per day for men and less than 2 drinks per day for women), drinking less than two and a half cups of coffee or five cups of tea per day, sun exposure of 30 minutes a day/5 days a week and vitamin D, 800 IU daily. Smoking cessation[11] and physical therapy[12] is also recommended.

Yoga and Osteoporosis

In a study of postmenopausal women without osteoporosis or osteopenia, weight bearing yoga decreased bone resorption. The experimental group (n=19) attended a 12-week weight-bearing yoga training, 3 days a week, 50 minutes a day while the control group (n=14) lived their normal lives. At the end of 12 weeks, the experimental group revealed decreased bone resorption and improved quality of life, compared to the control group[13].

In an observational cohort study involving twenty-six postmenopausal osteoporotic women over 55 years of age, the participants were randomized into a yoga group (n=13) and an exercise group. (n=13) The yoga group practiced yoga one hour twice a week for twelve weeks while the exercise group practiced classic osteoporosis exercises for one hour twice a week, for twelve weeks. The QUALEFFO test (Quality of life Questionnaire of the European foundation for Osteoporosis) revealed improvement in the exercise group in three parameters (pain, household activities and total score) while the yoga group showed improvement in all parameters. In conclusion, yoga was more effective in improving the quality of life in postmenopausal osteoporotic women[14].

Bone mineral density improved in spine, hips, and femur of 227 moderately and fully compliant patients, recruited in a study to check pre-yoga and 12 minute a day post-yoga BMD[15].

In another study recruited 30 postmenopausal females with osteoporosis (ages 45-62 years) with a dual-energy X-ray absorptiometry (DEXA) score of $\leq$-2.5. These participants underwent a 6 months fully supervised yoga session. At the end of the study, improvements in the T score of DEXA scan were noted[16].

Yoga also helps patients with osteoporosis improve their posture, balance, range of motion, strength, gait and coordination[17-19]. It also helps to decrease anxiety in these patients[20].

Conclusion

Yoga is effective and safe as an adjunct treatment of osteopenia and osteoporosis.

References

1. National Osteoporosis Foundation. Clinician's Guide to Prevention and Treatment of Osteoporosis. Washington, DC: National Osteoporosis Foundation; 2014.
2. Office of the Surgeon General (US) (2004) Bone health and osteoporosis: a report of the Surgeon General. Office of the Surgeon General (US), Rockville (MD).
3. National Osteoporosis Foundation. America's Bone Health: The State of Osteoporosis and Low Bone Mass in Our Nation. Washington, DC: National Osteoporosis Foundation; 2002.
4. Lewiecki EM, Laster AJ. Clinical review: clinical applications of vertebral fracture assessment by dual-energy x-ray absorptiometry. J Clin Endocrinol Metab. 2006;91(11):4215–4222. doi: 10.1210/jc.2006-1178.
5. U.S. Department of Health and Human Services. Bone Health and Osteoporosis: A Report of the Surgeon General. Rockville, Md.: U.S. Department of Health and Human Services, Office of the Surgeon General; 2004).
6. Cosman F, de Beur SJ, LeBoff MS, et al. Clinician's Guide to Prevention and Treatment of Osteoporosis. Osteoporosis International. 2014;25(10):2359-2381. doi:10.1007/s00198-014-2794-2.
7. Abrahamsen B, van Staa T, Ariely R, Olson M, Cooper C. Excess mortality following hip fracture: a systematic epidemiological review. Osteoporos Int. 2009;20(10):1633–1650. doi: 10.1007/s00198-009-0920-3.
8. World Health Organization. WHO scientific group on the assessment of osteoporosis at the primary health care level: summary meeting report. Brussels, Belgium; May 5–7, 2004. Geneva, Switzerland: World Health Organization; 2007.
9. Crandall CJ, Newberry SJ, Diamant A, et al. Comparative effectiveness of pharmacologic treatments to prevent fractures: an updated systematic review. Ann Intern Med. 2014;161(10):711–723.
10. Karinkanta S, Piirtola M, Sievänen H, Uusi-Rasi K, Kannus P. Physical therapy approaches to reduce fall and fracture risk among older adults. Nat Rev Endocrinol. 2010;6(7):396–407.
11. Krall EA, Dawson-Hughes B. Smoking increases bone loss and decreases intestinal calcium absorption. J Bone Miner Res. 1999;14:215–220. doi: 10.1359/jbmr.1999.14.2.215.
12. Choi M, Hector M. Effectiveness of intervention programs in preventing falls: a systematic review of recent 10 years and meta-analysis. J Am Med Dir Assoc. 2012;13(2):188.13–188.e21. doi: 10.1016/j.jamda.2011.04.022.

13. Phoosuwan M, Kritpet T, Yuktanandana P. The effects of weight bearing yoga training on the bone resorption markers of the postmenopausal women. J Med Assoc Thai. 2009;92(Suppl5):S102–8.
14. Tüzün S, Aktas I, Akarirmak U, Sipahi S, Tüzün F. Yoga might be an alternative training for the quality of life and balance in postmenopausal osteoporosis. Eur J Phys Rehabil Med. 2010;46:69–72.
15. Lu Y-H, Rosner B, Chang G, Fishman LM. Twelve-Minute Daily Yoga Regimen Reverses Osteoporotic Bone Loss. Topics in Geriatric Rehabilitation. 2016;32(2):81-87. doi:10.1097/TGR.0000000000000085.
16. Motorwala ZS, Kolke S, Panchal PY, Bedekar NS, Sancheti PK, Shyam A. Effects of Yogasanas on osteoporosis in postmenopausal women. Int J Yoga. 2016 Jan-Jun;9(1):44-8. doi: 10.4103/0973-6131.171717.
17. DiBenedetto M, Innes KE, Taylor AG, et al. Effect of a gentle Iyengar yoga program on gait in the elderly: an exploratory study. Arch Phys Med Rehabil. 2005;86:1830–1837.
18. Prado ET, Raso V, Scharlach RC, Kasse CA. Hatha yoga on body balance. Int J Yoga. 2014;7(2):133–137.
19. Grabara M, Szopa J. Effects of hatha yoga exercises on spine flexibility in women over 50 years old. J Phys Ther Sci. 2015;27:361–5.
20. Payne P, Crane-Godreau MA. Meditative movement for depression and anxiety. Front Psychiatry. 2013;4:71. 10.3389/fpsyt.2013.00071. eCollection 2013.

Polycystic Ovarian Syndrome

Polycystic ovary syndrome (PCOS), also defined as chronic hyperandrogenic anovulation syndrome, is the most prevalent female endocrine disorder[1,2]. It affects about 5-10% of reproductive-aged women[3]. Diagnosis is usually made using guidelines provided by the Endocrine Society[4].

Females with PCOS usually have menstrual abnormalities which include oligomenorrhea, amenorrhea, and prolonged erratic menstrual bleeding[5,6]. They may also have several cardio-metabolic co-morbid disorders such as dyslipidemia, endothelial dysfunction, hypertension, inflammation, obesity and subclinical atherosclerosis[7-12]. Insulin resistance makes them more at risk for impaired glucose tolerance and type 2 diabetes[13-16]. Because of hirsutism, irregular menses, acne, acanthosis nigricans, obesity, and infertility, they are at an increased risk for psychological distress, and often have anxiety, depression and diminished quality of life[17-19]. One study found the prevalence of emotional distress in these patients at 38% and depression at 21-46%[20-22]. Suicide attempts are also common in these patients[23,24].

Treatment is aimed at controlling individual symptoms such as infertility, hirsutism, acne or obesity. Medications used include oral contraceptives, metformin, prednisone, leuprolide, clomiphene, and spironolactone. Excessive hair may require removal with electrolysis. Complementary and alternative medicine is used by some patients with PCOS[25]. Yoga has also been tried.

Yoga and Polycystic Ovarian Syndrome

Yoga interventions have shown to be effective in reducing symptoms of stress and anxiety in patients with PCOS[26-28].

Twelve weeks of a holistic yoga program was compared to a matching physical activity program in ninety adolescent girls with PCOS. The yoga intervention group showed significant reduction in anxiety compared to the physical exercise group[26].

In a study of obese women, many with polycystic ovarian syndrome, using the Toronto Mindfulness Scale and the Perceived Stress Scale -10, researchers reported significantly lower stress at 16 weeks, in the mindfulness-based stress reduction (MBSR) group. The authors did not report the PCOS group results separately[27,28].

Conclusion

Anxiety and depression accompanying polycystic ovarian syndrome is reduced by yoga intervention.

References

1. Michelmore KF, Balen AH, Dunger DB, Vessey MP. Polycystic ovaries and associates; clinical and biochemical features in young women. Clin Endocrinol. 1999;51:779–86.
2. Chen X, Yang D, Mo Y, Li L, Chen Y, Huang Y. Prevalence of polycystic ovary syndrome in unselected women from southern China. Eur J Obstet Gynecol Reprod Biol. 2008;139:59–64.
3. Raja-Khan N, Legro RS. Diagnosis and management of polycystic ovary syndrome. J Clin Outcomes Manage. 2005;12(4):218–227.
4. Legro RS; Arslanian SA; Ehrmann DA; Hoeger KM; Murad MH; Pasquali R; Welt CK. Diagnosis and treatment of polycystic ovary syndrome: An Endocrine Society clinical practice guideline. J Clin Endocrinol Metab. 2013; 98(12):4565-92 (ISSN: 1945-7197.
5. (Farquhar C. Introduction and history of polycystic ovary syndrome. In: Kovacs G, Norman R, editors. Polycystic Ovary Syndrome. 2nd ed. Cambridge, UK: Cambridge University Press; 2007. pp. 4–24.
6. Sirmans SM, Pate KA. Epidemiology, diagnosis, and management of polycystic ovary syndrome. Clinical Epidemiology. 2014;6:1-13. doi:10.2147/CLEP.S37559.
7. Legro RS, et al. Prevalence and predictors of dyslipidemia in women with polycystic ovary syndrome. Am J Med. 2001;111(8):607–13.
8. Ehrmann DA. Polycystic ovary syndrome. N Engl J Med. 2005;352(12):1223–36.
9. Lo JC, et al. Epidemiology and adverse cardiovascular risk profile of diagnosed polycystic ovary syndrome. J Clin Endocrinol Metab. 2006;91(4):1357–63.
10. Meyer C, McGrath BP, Teede HJ. Overweight women with polycystic ovary syndrome have evidence of subclinical cardiovascular disease. J Clin Endocrinol Metab. 2005;90(10):5711–6.
11. Shroff R, et al. Young obese women with polycystic ovary syndrome have evidence of early coronary atherosclerosis. J Clin Endocrinol Metab. 2007;92(12):4609–14.
12. Gonzalez F, et al. Evidence of proatherogenic inflammation in polycystic ovary syndrome. Metabolism. 2009;58(7):954–62.
13. Legro RS, et al. Prevalence and predictors of risk for type 2 diabetes mellitus and impaired glucose tolerance in polycystic ovary syndrome: a

prospective, controlled study in 254 affected women. J Clin Endocrinol Metab. 1999;84(1):165–9.

14. Legro RS, et al. Changes in glucose tolerance over time in women with polycystic ovary syndrome: a controlled study. J Clin Endocrinol Metab. 2005;90(6):3236–42.

15. Ehrmann DA, et al. Prevalence of impaired glucose tolerance and diabetes in women with polycystic ovary syndrome. Diabetes Care. 1999;22(1):141–6.

16. Karakas SE, Kim K, Duleba AJ. Determinants of impaired fasting glucose vs. glucose intolerance in polycystic ovary syndrome. Diabetes Care. 2010;33(4):887–93.

17. Himelein MJ, Thatcher SS. Depression and body image among women with polycystic ovary syndrome. J Health Psychol. 2006;11(4):613–25.

18. Barnard L, et al. Quality of life and psychological well being in polycystic ovary syndrome. Hum Reprod. 2007;22(8):2279–86.

19. Bishop SC, Basch S, Futterweit W. Polycystic ovary syndrome, depression, and affective disorders. Endocr Pract. 2009;15(5):475–82.

20. Hollinrake E, et al. Increased risk of depressive disorders in women with polycystic ovary syndrome. Fertil Steril. 2007;87(6):1369–76.

21. Adali E, et al. The relationship between clinico-biochemical characteristics and psychiatric distress in young women with polycystic ovary syndrome. J Int Med Res. 2008;36(6):1188–96.

22. Benson S, et al. Disturbed stress responses in women with polycystic ovary syndrome. Psychoneuroendocrinology. 2009;34(5):727–35.

23. Mansson M, et al. Women with polycystic ovary syndrome are often depressed or anxious--a case control study. Psychoneuroendocrinology. 2008;33(8):1132–8.

24. Deeks AA, Gibson-Helm ME, Teede HJ. Anxiety and depression in polycystic ovary syndrome: A comprehensive investigation. Fertil Steril. 2010;93:2421–3.

25. Amini L, Tehranian N, Movahedin M, Ramezani Tehrani F, Ziaee S. Antioxidants and management of polycystic ovary syndrome in Iran: A systematic review of clinical trials. Iranian Journal of Reproductive Medicine. 2015;13(1):1-8.

26. Ram Nidhi, Venkatram Padmalatha, Raghuram Nagarathna, Ram Amritanshu. Effect of holistic yoga program on anxiety symptoms in adolescent girls with polycystic ovarian syndrome: A randomized control trial. Int J Yoga. 2012 Jul-Dec; 5(2): 112–117. doi: 10.4103/0973-6131.98223.

27. Nazia Raja-Khan, Katrina Agito, Julie Shah, Christy M. Stetter, Theresa S. Gustafson, Holly Socolow, Allen R. Kunselman, Diane K. Reibel, Richard S. Legro. Mindfulness-Based Stress Reduction for Overweight/Obese Women with and Without Polycystic Ovary Syndrome: Design and Methods of a Pilot Randomized Controlled Trial. Contemp Clin Trials. 2015 Mar; 41: 287–297.

28. Raja-Khan N, Agito K, Shah J, et al. Mindfulness-Based Stress Reduction in Women with Overweight or Obesity: A Randomized

Clinical Trial. Obesity (Silver Spring, Md). 2017;25(8):1349-1359. doi:10.1002/oby.21910.

Post Stroke Rehabilitation

Stroke is a common disorder, affecting about 15 million people worldwide each year[1]. A major percentage of stroke survivors (80%-90%) are left with some type of disability[2,3]. It is the third major cause of loss of disability-adjusted life years among 291 adverse health conditions worldwide[4] These patients are also burdened with a significant decrease in their quality of life[5]. Post stroke rehabilitation helps improved functionality and reduces long-term disability[6]. Co-morbidities are common in stroke patients, the top three being hypertension, cardiovascular diseases and diabetes mellitus[7,8]. Post-stroke depression is also a common emotional disorder in these patients[9]. Following a stroke, the patient is usually transferred to an inpatient rehabilitation facility, a skilled nursing facility or a long-term acute care hospital. Some are discharged home. Post-stroke rehabilitation is continued following hospital discharge[10]. Rehabilitation is aimed at recovery of function and cognition to the maximum level achievable, allowing stroke survivors to engage in meaningful life activities. Post-stroke rehabilitation involves many different techniques, mostly based on motor learning to induce neural plasticiticity[11]. Complementary and alternative medicine therapies have also been used in stroke rehabilitation[12]. Yoga practice has also been tried in this physical and mental rehabilitation process[13].

Yoga and Post Stroke Rehabilitation

Published studies, although limited, suggest that yoga is a useful tool for the rehabilitation process after stroke.

In a study involving eight female participants, with a mean age of 84 years, and 8 control participants, 5 women and 3 men, average age 81.3 years, an 8-week, 80-minute biweekly Kripalu yoga class was noted to improve postural control, mobility, and gait speed. The researchers suggested that these benefits should also be possible in post-stroke patients with yoga[14].

In another study by Garrett and group, nine post stroke patients underwent a 10-week yoga training program. The patients reported improved sensation, feeling calmer and becoming connected to a new body. Yoga practice also resulted in improvement in strength, range of motion, and walking ability[15] and balance[16].

In a small study involving four post-stroke patients, functionality was monitored using the Berg Balance Scale and the Timed Movement Battery. The patients underwent yoga practice for 1.5-hour yoga sessions, 2 times per week, for 8 weeks, in their home. Improvements in mobility and balance were noted[17]. Improved balance with yoga was also reported in another study[18].

Schmid and associates[19] recruited 47 patients with chronic stroke and randomized them to a therapeutic-yoga group (n=37) or a wait-list control group (n=10). After 16 sessions of therapeutic yoga (twice a week/8 weeks) they reported that the yoga group had significant improvements in pain, neck range of motion (ROM), hip passive ROM, upper extremity strength, and 6-minute walk scores.

Quality of life, related to motor functions and memory/emotions, also improved in the yoga group, in a randomized controlled trial after a 10-week yoga intervention (n = 11) compared to the group with no treatment (n = 11)[20].

A meta-analysis (five randomized controlled clinical trials, four single case studies and one qualitative research study) documented an overall improvement in cognition, mood, and balance and reductions in stress in post-stroke patients practicing yoga[21]. Improvements in depression and anxiety with yoga were also noticed in another meta-analysis[22].

Conclusion

Although properly designed rigorous studies on the role of yoga in post-stroke rehabilitation are scant, available evidence based data suggests a potentially beneficial role.

References

1. Mackay J, Mensah GA: The Atlas of Heart Disease and Stroke. Geneva: World Health Organization, 2002.; Chong JY, Sacco RL: Epidemiology of stroke in young adults: race/ethnic differences. J Thromb Thrombolysis, 2005, 20: 77–83., WHO 2015.
2. Go AS, Mozaffarian D, Roger VL, et al. American Heart Association Statistics Committee and Stroke Statistics Subcommittee: heart disease

and stroke statistics—2013 update: a report from the American Heart Association. Circulation, 2013, 127: 6–245.

3. Silva SM, Corrêa FI, Faria CDC de M, Buchalla CM, Silva PF da C, Corrêa JCF. Evaluation of post-stroke functionality based on the International Classification of Functioning, Disability, and Health: a proposal for use of assessment tools. Journal of Physical Therapy Science. 2015;27(6):1665-1670. doi:10.1589/jpts.27.1665.

4. Murray CJ, Vos T, Lozano R, et al. Disability-adjusted life years (DALYs) for 291 diseases and injuries in 21 regions, 1990–2010: a systematic analysis for the Global Burden of Disease Study 2010. Lancet, 2012, 380: 2197–2223.

5. Saposnik G and C. J. Estol, "Translational research: from observational studies to health policy: how a cohort study can help improve outcomes after stroke," Stroke, vol. 42, no. 12, pp. 3336–3337, 2011.

6. Langhorne P., Bernhardt J., Kwakkel G. (2011). Stroke rehabilitation. Lancet 377, 1693–1702. 10.1016/S0140-6736(11)60325-5.

7. Roth EJ. Heart disease in patients with stroke. Part II: Impact and implications for rehabilitation. Archives of physical medicine and rehabilitation. 1994;75(1):94–94.

8. Liu M, Tsuji T, Tsujiuchi K, Chino N. Comorbidities in stroke patients as assessed with a newly developed comorbidity scale. Am J Phys Med Rehabil. 1999;78:416–24.

9. Gaete JM1, Bogousslavsky J. Post-stroke depression. Expert Rev Neurother. 2008 Jan;8(1):75-92.

10. Carolee J. Winstein, Joel Stein, Ross Arena, et al. Guidelines for Adult Stroke Rehabilitation and Recovery. A Guideline for Healthcare Professionals from the American Heart Association/American Stroke Association. Stroke. 2016;47:e98-e169.

11. Brewer L, Horgan F, Hickey A, Williams D. Stroke rehabilitation: recent advances and future therapies. QJM. 2013;106(1):11–25.

12. Sun F, Wang J, Wen X. Acupuncture in stroke rehabilitation: Literature retrieval based on international databases. Neural Regeneration Research. 2012;7(15):1192-1199. doi:10.3969/j.issn.1673-5374.2012.15.011.

13. Bastille JV, Gill-Body KM. A yoga-based exercise program for people with chronic poststroke hemiparesis. Phys Ther. 2004;84:33–48.

14. Zettergren KK, Lubeski JM, Viverito JM. Effects of a yoga program on postural control, mobility, and gait speed in community-living older adults: a pilot study. J Geriatr Phys Ther. 2011 Apr-Jun;34(2):88-94.

15. Garrett R, Immink MA, Hillier S. Becoming connected: The lived experience of yoga participation after stroke. Disabil Rehabil. 2011:1–12.

16. Bastille JV, Gill-Body KM. A yoga-based exercise program for people with chronic poststroke hemiparesis. Phys Ther. 2004; 84:33–48.

17. Bastille JV, Gill-Body KM. A yoga-based exercise program for people with chronic poststroke hemiparesis. Phys Ther. 2004;84:33–48.

18. Schmid A. A, Marieke Van Puymbroeck, Peter A. Altenburger et al. Poststroke Balance Improves with Yoga. A Pilot Study. Stroke. 2012; 43: 2402-2407.

19. Schmid AA, Miller KK, Van Puymbroeck M, DeBaun-Sprague E. Yoga leads to multiple physical improvements after stroke, a pilot study. Complement Ther Med. 2014 Dec;22(6):994-1000. doi: 10.1016/j.ctim.2014.09.005. Epub 2014 Oct 7.

20. Immink MA, Hillier S, Petkov J. Randomized controlled trial of yoga for chronic poststroke hemiparesis: motor function, mental health, and quality of life outcomes. Top Stroke Rehabil. 2014 May-Jun;21(3):256-71. doi: 10.1310/tsr2103-256.

21. Asimina Lazaridou, Phaethon Philbrook, and Aria A. Tzika. Yoga and Mindfulness as Therapeutic Interventions for Stroke Rehabilitation: A Systematic Review. Evidence-Based Complementary and Alternative Medicine. Volume 2013.

22. Thayabaranathan T, Andrew NE1, Immink MA et al. Determining the potential benefits of yoga in chronic stroke care: a systematic review and meta-analysis. Top Stroke Rehabil. 2017 May;24(4):279-287. doi: 10.1080/10749357.2016.1277481. Epub 2017 Jan 19.

Pregnancy Disorders

Several medical problems can occur during and after pregnancy. These include anemia, gestational diabetes mellitus, hypertension, hyperemesis gravidarum, obesity and urinary tract infection. Depression may also occur. It is estimated that prenatal depression occurs in about 20% of the teenage pregnant women[1] and in about 10–25% of adult pregnant women[2].

Symptoms of depression during pregnancy include low or sad mood, loss of interest in fun activities, changes in appetite, sleep, and energy, and problems with thinking, concentrating, and making decisions. There may be feelings of worthlessness, shame, or guilt, and thoughts that life is not worth living[3]. Prenatal depression often leads to postpartum depression and paternal depression in the father. The neonates are more likely to be born premature, with lower birth weight and lower Apgar and Brazelton scores[4].

Pharmacological treatment is usually avoided but may be used if needed[5]. Non-pharmacological treatments for depression, such as cognitive behavioral therapy[6,7] and complementary treatments[8] are usually safe during pregnancy and can help reduce symptoms of depression. Yoga has been successfully tried in these women, especially to relieve depression[9].

Yoga and Pregnancy Disorders

Several studies support the acceptability of prenatal yoga among women seeking treatment for antenatal depression[10-13].

In a meta-analysis of six trials (three were randomized controlled trials and three were controlled trials) Curtis and group noted several improvements with gentle yoga performed during pregnancy. These benefits were seen in a variety of pregnancy, labor, and birth outcomes[14].

In a more recent meta-analysis[15], involving six randomly controlled trials with 375 pregnant women, depression was documented by their scores on Structured Clinical Interview for DSM-IV and the Center for Epidemiological Studies Depression Scale. Yoga practice significantly reduced depression when compared with comparison groups (e.g., standard prenatal care, standard antenatal exercises, social support, etc.).

Mindfulness practice and yoga have been shown to decrease the total labor time, perception of pain during labor, and physical discomfort during pregnancy. Yoga patients also experience a significant reduction in stress and anxiety[16-18].

Conclusion

Tailored gentle yoga during pregnancy not only helps reduce depression, but also positively affects other pregnancy related outcomes.

References

1. Abajobir AA, Maravilla JC, Alati R, Najman JM. A systematic review and meta-analysis of the association between unintended pregnancy and perinatal depression. J Affect Disord. 2016;192:56–63.
2. Accortt EE, Cheadle AC, Schetter CD. Prenatal depression and adverse birth outcomes: An updated systematic review. Matern Child Health. 2015;19:1306–1337.
3. https://www.cdc.gov/reproductivehealth/maternalinfanthealth/pregcompli cations.htm - accessed 11/27/17.
4. Field T. Prenatal Depression Risk Factors, Developmental Effects and Interventions: A Review. Journal of pregnancy and child health. 2017;4(1):301. doi:10.4172/2376-127X.1000301.
5. Accortt EE, Cheadle ACD, Schetter CD. Prenatal Depression and Adverse Birth Outcomes: An Updated Systematic Review. Maternal and child health journal. 2015;19(6):1306-1337. doi:10.1007/s10995-014-1637-2.
6. Burns A, Heather O, Baxter H, Bennert K, Wiles N, Ramchandani P, et al. A pilot randomised controlled trial of cognitive behavioural therapy for antenatal depression. BMC Psychiatry. 2013;13(1):33.
7. O'Mahen H, Himle JA, Fedock G, Henshaw E, Flynn H. A pilot randomized controlled trial of cognitive behavioral therapy for perinatal depression adapted for women with low incomes. Depression and Anxiety. 2013;30(7):679–687.
8. Field T, Diego M, Hernandez-Reif M, Medina L, Delgado J, Hernandez A. Yoga and massage therapy reduce prenatal depression and prematurity. Journal of bodywork and movement therapies. 2012;16(2):204–209.
9. Cynthia L. Battle, Lisa A. Uebelacker, Susanna R. Magee, Kaeli A. Sutton, Ivan W. Miller. Potential for prenatal yoga to serve as an intervention to treat depression during pregnancy. Womens' Health Issues. 2015 Mar-Apr; 25(2): 134–141. doi: 10.1016/j.whi.2014.12.003.

10. Sun YC, Hung YC, Chang Y, Kuo SC. Effects of a prenatal yoga programme on the discomforts of pregnancy and maternal childbirth self-efficacy in Taiwan. Midwifery. 2010;26(6): e31–6. 35.

11. Battle CL, Uebelacker LA, Howard M, Castaneda M. Prenatal yoga and depression during pregnancy. Birth. 2010;37(4):353–4.

12. Chuntharapat S, Petpichetchian W, Hatthakit U. Yoga during pregnancy: effects on maternal comfort, labor pain and birth outcomes. Complement Ther Clin Pract. 2008;14(2):105–15.

13. Narendran S, Nagarathna R, Narendran V, Gunasheela S, Nagendra HR. Efficacy of yoga on pregnancy outcome. J Altern Complement Med. 2005;11(2):237–44.

14. Curtis K, Weinrib A, Katz J. Systematic Review of Yoga for Pregnant Women: Current Status and Future Directions. Evidence-based Complementary and Alternative Medicine□: eCAM. 2012;2012:715942. doi:10.1155/2012/715942.

15. Hong Gong, Chenxu Ni, Xiaoliang Shen, Tengyun Wu, Chunlei Jiang. Yoga for prenatal depression: a systematic review and meta-analysis. BMC Psychiatry. 2015; 15: 14.

16. Chuntharapat S, Petpichetchian W, Hatthakit U. Yoga during pregnancy: effects on maternal comfort, labor pain and birth outcomes. Complement Ther Clin Pract. 2008;14(2):105–15.

17. Beddoe AE, Lee KA. Mind-body interventions during pregnancy. J Obstet Gynecol Neonatal Nurs. 2008;37(2):165–75.

18. Satyapriyaa M, Nagendraa HR, Nagarathnaa R, Padmalathab V. Effects of integrated yoga on stress and heart rate variability in pregnant women. Int J Obstet Gynecol. 2009;104(3):218–222.

Post-Traumatic Stress Disorder (PTSD)

Posttraumatic stress disorder (PTSD) results from being exposed to a traumatic event. It is characterized by persistent re-experiencing, avoidance, numbing, and hyperarousal symptoms following the experiencing, witnessing, or confrontation with actual or potential death, serious physical injury, or a threat to physical integrity[1].

Posttraumatic stress disorder is a common disorder in the general population[2,3], with the life time prevalence approaching 7.8 %[4]. PTSD, along with other service-related mental disorders occur in high rates in the armed foreeces[5,6]. It is more common in women, both in the general population[7] as well in veterans[8]. It is often accompanied by other psychiatric abnormalities such mood disturbances, anxiety, alcohol use/dependence, drug abuse/dependence, conduct disorders and suicide ideation and attempts[9,10]. They also have more co-morbid physical health problems, including obesity, low back pain, smoking, irritable bowel syndrome, fibromyalgia, chronic pelvic pain, polycystic ovary disease, asthma, cervical cancer, and stroke[11].

These patients exhibit high sympathetic activity coupled with low parasympathetic cardiac control and respiratory abnormalities[12]. Treatment consists of pharmacotherapy and psychotherapy. Side effects from medications are not uncommon[13].

Many patients and healthcare providers use complementary and alternative medicine for the adjunct treatment of PTSD[14]. Yoga is also commonly used by these patients[15,16].

Yoga and PTSD

People exposed to stress and at risk for developing PTSD benefit from yoga. A week of yoga a month after a calamity (floods in India) reduced feelings of sadness, and helped prevent increased anxiety[17].

In an analysis of 10 studies to examine the efficacy of yoga therapy as a complementary treatment for psychiatric disorders such as schizophrenia, depression, anxiety, and posttraumatic stress disorder, Cabral and his group found that yoga-based interventions have a statistically significant beneficial effect as an adjunct treatment for major psychiatric disorders[18].

Telles and his associates reviewed 8 studies on PTSD following natural disasters or combat and terrorism. Yoga practice (1 week to six months) reduced symptoms of PTSD in all groups exposed to a traumatic event[19].

Mitchell and associates conducted a randomized controlled trial in 38 women with current full or subthreshold PTSD symptoms. The yoga group was given a 12-session Kripalu-based yoga intervention. When compared to the assessment control group, yoga intervention participants showed decreases in re-experiencing and hyperarousal symptoms[20].

In a study of 64 women with chronic, treatment-resistant PTSD, researchers randomized them to of trauma-informed yoga (10 sessions,1 hour per session/week) or supportive women's health education. At the end of the study, they reported that yoga significantly reduced PTSD symptomatology. According to the researchers, this benefit was comparable to other psychotherapeutic and psychopharmacologic approaches[21].

In another study, PTSD females, aged 18-65 years old, were exposed to yoga practice (12 Kripalu-based Hatha yoga sessions of 75 minutes each). At the end of the study, 69% of participants in the yoga group reported a decrease in symptoms, while 80% of the control group reported their symptoms as same or increased. The yoga group was also able to cope better with their PTSD symptoms (92% compared to 9% in the control group)[22].

Conclusion

Yoga modalities appear to significantly improve symptoms in patients with PTSD. Yoga helps downgrade the stress response. It also helps improve comorbid depression and anxiety symptoms, in these patients.

References

1. American Psychiatric Association. Diagnostic and statistical manual of mental disorders-text revision (DSM-IV-TR) Washington, DC: American Psychiatric Press; 2000.

2. Kessler RC CW. Prevalence, severity, and comorbidity of 12-month DSM-IV disorders in the national comorbidity survey replication. Arch Gen Psychiatry 2005;62:617–627,

3. Stein MB, McQuaid JR, Pedrelli P, Lenox R, McCahill ME. Posttraumatic stress disorder in the primary care medical setting. Gen Hosp Psychiatry 2000;22:261–269.

4. Kessler RC, Sonnega A, Bromet E, Hughes M, Nelson CB. Posttraumatic stress disorder in the National Comorbidity Survey. Archives of General Psychiatry. 1995;52:1048–1060.

5. Seal KH, Metzler TJ, Gima KS, et al. Trends and risk factors for mental health diagnoses among Iraq and Afghanistan veterans using Department of Veterans Affairs health care, 2002–2008. Am J Public Helath 2009;99:1651–1658.

6. Seal KH Bertenthal B, Miner CR, Marmar C. Bringing the war back home: mental health disorders among 103 788 us veterans returning from Iraq and Afghanistan seen at Department of Veterans Affairs facilities. Arch Intern Med 2007;167:476–42.

7. Mitchell K, Mazzeo S, Schlesinger M, Brewerton T, Smith B. Comorbidity of partial and subthreshold PTSD among men and women with eating disorders in the National Comorbidity Survey-Replication study. Int J Eat Disord 2012;45:307–315.

8. Freedy J, Magruder K, Mainous A, Frueh B, Geesey M, Carnemolla M. gender differences in traumatic event exposure and mental health among veteran primary care patients. Mil Med 2010;175:750–758.

9. Kessler RC, Chiu WT, Demler O, Merikangas KR, Walters EE. Prevalence, severity, and comorbidity of 12-month DSM-IV disorders in the National Comorbidity Survey Replication. Archives of General Psychiatry. 2005;62:617–627.

10. Cougle JR, Keough ME, Riccardi CJ, Sachs-Ericsson N. Anxiety disorders and suicidality in the National Comorbidity Survey-Replication. Journal of Psychiatric Research. 2009;43:825–829.

11. Dobie DJ, Kivlahan DR, Maynard C, et al. Posttraumatic stress disorder in female veterans: association with self-reported health problems and functional impairment. Arch Intern Med 2004;164:394–400.

12. Blechert J, Michael T, Grossman P, Lajtman M, Wilhelm FH. Autonomic and respiratory characteristics of posttraumatic stress disorder and panic disorder. Psychosom Med. 2007;69:935–943. doi: 10.1097/PSY.0b013e31815a8f6b.

13. Libby DJ, Pilver CE, Desai R. Complementary and alternative medicine use among individuals with posttraumatic stress disorder. Psychol Trauma Theory Res Pract Policy 2013;5:277–285.

14. Libby DJ, Pilver CE, Desai R. Complementary and alternative medicine use among individuals with posttraumatic stress disorder. Psychol Trauma Theory Res Pract Policy 2013;5:277–285.

15. Barnes PM, Bloom B, Nahin RL. Complementary and alternative medicine use among adults and children: United States, 2007. Natl Health Stat Rep 2008; 1–23.

16. Duan-Porter W, Coeytaux RR, McDuffie J, et al. Evidence Map of Yoga for Depression, Anxiety, and Posttraumatic Stress Disorder. Journal of physical activity & health. 2016;13(3):281-288. doi:10.1123/jpah.2015-0027.

17. Telles S, Singh N, Joshi M, Balkrishna A. Post traumatic stress symptoms and heart rate variability in Bihar flood survivors following yoga: a randomized controlled study. BMC Psychiatry. 2010;10:18. doi:10.1186/1471-244X-10-18.

18. Cabral P, Meyer HB, Ames D. Effectiveness of yoga therapy as a complementary treatment for major psychiatric disorders: a meta-analysis. Prim Care Companion CNS Disord. 2011;13(4):PCC.10r01068.

19. Telles S, Singh N, Balkrishna A. Managing mental health disorders resulting from trauma through yoga: a review. Depression Research and Treatment. 2012;2012:9 pages.40151.

20. Mitchell KS, Dick AM, DiMartino DM, et al. A pilot study of a randomized controlled trial of yoga as an intervention for PTSD symptoms in women. J Trauma Stress. 2014;27:121–128. doi: 10.1002/jts.21903.

21. van der Kolk BA, Stone L, West J, et al. Yoga as an adjunctive treatment for posttraumatic stress disorder: a randomized controlled trial. J Clin Psychiatry. 2014;75:e559–e565. doi: 10.4088/JCP.13m08561.

22. Reddy S, Dick AM, Gerber MR, Mitchell K. The Effect of a Yoga Intervention on Alcohol and Drug Abuse Risk in Veteran and Civilian Women with Posttraumatic Stress Disorder. Journal of Alternative and Complementary Medicine. 2014;20(10):750-756. doi:10.1089/acm.2014.0014.

Restless Leg Syndrome (RLS)

Restless leg syndrome (RLS) is characterized by uncomfortable leg sensations, usually at sleep onset, with an irresistible urge to move the legs. These sensations include itching, crawling, creeping, and tingling in the legs. These are temporarily relieved with leg movements. The prevalence rate of restless leg syndrome ranges from 3.9% to 15% in the general population[1]. It is twice as common in women[2]. It is often associated with other conditions, such as obesity[3], cardiovascular diseases[4], arthritis[5] and uremia[6]. RLS may occur during pregnancy and usually disappears after delivery[7]. Depression is also common in these patients[8]. Pathophysiological mechanisms are unclear but may be related to dysfunction of the iron metabolism[9] and/or dysregulation of the dopamine system[10].

Treatment consists of dopaminergic agents such as pramipexole and ropinirole[11] and antidepressants[12.] Nonpharmacological approaches, include better sleep hygiene, avoiding substances or medications that may exacerbate RLS[13] and exercise[14].

Yoga and Restless Leg Syndrome

In a pilot study, 13 non-smoking women were enrolled and 10 finished the study. They participated in a gentle Iyengar yoga program for 8 weeks. Pre- and post-intervention, patients were evaluated for RLS symptoms and symptom severity (International RLS Scale and RLS ordinal scale), sleep quality (Medical Outcomes Study Sleep Scale), mood (Profile of Mood States), and perceived stress (Perceived Stress Scale). At the end of the study, participants reported striking reductions in RLS symptoms and symptom severity[15].

Conclusion

According to this small pilot study, yoga may be effective in reducing RLS symptoms, symptom severity and perceived stress. Yoga also helps improve the mood and sleep in women with RLS.

References

1. Ohayon M. M., O'hara R., Vitiello M. V. (2012). Epidemiology of restless legs syndrome: a synthesis of the literature. Sleep Med. Rev. 16 283–295.10.1016/j.smrv.2011.05.002.
2. Ohayon MM, O'Hara R, Vitiello MV. Epidemiology of Restless Legs Syndrome: A Synthesis of the Literature. Sleep Medicine Reviews. 2012;16(4):283-295. doi:10.1016/j.smrv.2011.05.002.
3. Gao X, Schwarzschild MA, Wang H, Ascherio A. Obesity and restless legs syndrome in men and women. Neurology. 2009;72:1255–1261.
4. Winkelman JW, Shahar E, Sharief I, Gottlieb DJ. Association of restless legs syndrome and cardiovascular disease in the Sleep Heart Health Study. Neurology. 2008;70:35–42.
5. Chen NH, Chuang LP, Yang CT, Kushida CA, Hsu SC, Wang PC, Lin SW, Chou YT, Chen RS, Li HY, Lai SC. The prevalence of restless legs syndrome in Taiwanese adults. Psychiatry Clin Neurosci. 2010;64:170–178.
6. Callaghan N. Restless legs syndrome and uremic neuropathy. Neurology. 1966;16:359–361.
7. Picchietti DL, Hensley JG, Bainbridge JL, et al. Consensus clinical practice guidelines for the diagnosis and treatment of restless legs syndrome/Willis-Ekbom disease during pregnancy and lactation. Sleep Med Rev 2015;22:64–77.
8. Lee HB, Hening WA, Allen RP, Kalaydjian AE, Earley CJ, Eaton WW, Lyketsos CG. Restless legs syndrome is associated with DSM-IV major depressive disorder and panic disorder in the community. J Neuropsychiatry Clin Neurosci. 2008;20:101–105.
9. Dauvilliers Y., Winkelmann J. (2013). Restless legs syndrome: update on pathogenesis. Curr. Opin. Pulm. Med. 19 594–600. 10.1097/MCP.0b013e328365ab07.
10. Swanson J. M., Kinsbourne M., Nigg J., Lanphear B., Stefanatos G. A., Volkow N., et al. (2007). Etiologic subtypes of attention-deficit/hyperactivity disorder: brain imaging, molecular genetic and environmental factors and the dopamine hypothesis. Neuropsychol. Rev. 17 39–59. 10.1007/s11065-007-9019-9.
11. Silber M. H., Becker P. M., Earley C., Garcia-Borreguero D., Ondo W. G., Medical Advisory Board of the Willis-Ekbom Disease Foundation (2013). Willis-Ekbom disease foundation revised consensus statement on the management of restless legs syndrome. Mayo Clin. Proc. 88 977–986.10.1016/j.mayocp.2013.06.016.
12. Mackie S., Winkelman J. W. (2015). Long-term treatment of restless legs syndrome (RLS): an approach to management of worsening symptoms, loss of efficacy, and augmentation. CNS Drugs 29 351–357. 10.1007/s40263-015-0250-2.
13. Guo S, Huang J, Jiang H, et al. Restless Legs Syndrome: From Pathophysiology to Clinical Diagnosis and Management. Frontiers in Aging Neuroscience. 2017;9:171. doi:10.3389/fnagi.2017.00171.

14. Aukerman MM, Aukerman D, Bayard M, Tudiver F, Thorp L, Bailey B. Exercise and restless legs syndrome: a randomized controlled trial. J Am Board Fam Med. 2006;19:487–493.

15. Innes KE, Selfe TK, Agarwal P, Williams K, Flack KL. Efficacy of an Eight-Week Yoga Intervention on Symptoms of Restless Legs Syndrome (RLS): A Pilot Study. Journal of Alternative and Complementary Medicine. 2013;19(6):527-535. doi:10.1089/acm.2012.0330.

Rheumatoid Arthritis

Rheumatoid arthritis (RA) is a chronic systemic inflammatory disease of unknown cause. It affects over 1.3 million Americans and as many as 1% of the worldwide population[1].

Diagnosis is usually based on symptoms of persistent symmetric polyarthritis, including that of hands, progressing to difficulty performing activities of daily living. Morning stiffness usually lasts 30 minutes or longer, with symptoms being of more than six months duration. Patients may also complain of low grade fever, fatigue, loss of appetite and weight loss. They may be depressed. Signs include joint stiffness and swelling, tenderness, pain and restriction of motion, and rheumatoid nodules. Rheumatoid arthritis may be seropositive (positive for rheumatoid factor and/or anti-cyclic citrullinated peptide) or seronegative (negative for either antibody). Overall, these patients have a lower life-span by about 10-15 years[2].

Treatment consists of pharmacology with nonbiologic disease-modifying antirheumatic drugs (DMARDS) (such as hydroxycholoroquine. sulfasalazine, and methotrexate) and biologic tumor necrosis factor (TNF)–inhibiting DMARDs (such as rituximab). Other drugs like corticosteroids, nonsteroidal anti-inflammatory drugs (NSAIDs) and analgesics are often used. Non-pharmacologic treatments include heat and cold therapies, orthotics and splints, therapeutic exercise and occupational therapy. Adaptive equipment may be given to these patients. Surgical treatments include synovectomy, tenosynovectomy, tendon realignment, reconstructive surgery or arthroplasty and arthrodesis. Complementary and alternative medicine is also commonly used by rheumatoid arthritis patients[3]. Yoga also appears to help patients with rheumatoid arthritis[4].

Yoga and Rheumatoid Arthritis

Psychological distress in patients with rheumatoid arthritis was improved by mindfulness based stress reduction (MBSR) in 31 patients, with a control of 32 patients, after 6 months. There was also some improvement in depressive symptoms in the treated group[5]. A decrease in depressive symptoms was also reported in a later study[6].

In a matched paired controlled study, 20 volunteers with RA were allocated to yoga (n = 10) or control (n = 10) groups. The yoga group participated in a yoga session for 2 hours, 5 days a week for 3 weeks. This was followed by weekly 2-hour sessions over the next 3 months. Home practice for 10-30 minutes was done on the remaining days. At the end of 3 months, using the Stanford Health Assessment Questionnaire Disability Index, and psychological assessment using the General Health Questionnaire, researchers noted improvement in the left-hand grip strength in the yoga group compared to the control group[7]. Improvement in hand grip strength with yoga was also noted in 20 patients in the yoga group when compared to 20 patients in the control group, in another study[8].

In a trial of 47 patients with rheumatoid arthritis, randomization resulted in 21 in the yoga group and 21 in the control group. The yoga group underwent 12 sessions of yoga over a period of 6 weeks (2 sessions per week of 1 hour each). Significant improvements in tender joint count, swollen joint count, DAS 28 (disease activity scores using 28 joint count), and HAQ (Health Assessment Questionnaire) were observed in the yoga group[9].

Twenty postmenopausal women (ages between 45 and 75 years) were allocated to yoga (n = 11) or control (n = 9) groups. Yoga sessions were conducted over a 10-week interval with 3 classes per week with each class lasting for 75 minutes for 10 weeks. At the end of the study, there were improvements noted in pain in the yoga group. Balance was better and depression symptoms were decreased in these patients[10].

In a pilot study involving eight young adults with rheumatoid arthritis, six-week, biweekly yoga program resulted in significant improvements in pain, pain disability, depression, mental health, vitality, and self-efficacy[11].

A short study with 64 patients with rheumatoid arthritis also revealed benefits with yoga. The study lasted one week, during which time two yoga sessions were held each day and each session lasted for 2:30 hours. At the end of the study, the female participants note improvement in dressing, arising, and walking, while in the male participants, a significant improvement was observed in dressing, walking and grip strength[12].

In a study of 26 female patients (mean age =28 years) with 11 in the yoga group and 15 in the usual care waitlist group, the effects on the health-related quality of life (HRQOL) were reviewed. After 6-weeks of twice/week Iyengar yoga, and after 2 months following treatment, Evans and group noted significantly greater improvement on standardized measures of HRQOL in the yoga group. The patients also reported lesser pain disability, improved general health, mood, decreased fatigue. They also had better acceptance of chronic pain and self-efficacy regarding pain at post treatment[13].

Conclusion

Yoga should be considered as an add-on therapy in patients with rheumatoid arthritis.

References

1. https://www.rheumatoidarthritis.org/ra/facts-and-statistics/.-accessed 11/1/17.
2. http://www.arthritis.org/about-arthritis/types/rheumatoid-arthritis/symptoms.php - accessed 1/20/18.
3. Efthimiou P, Kukar M, MacKenzie CR. Complementary and Alternative Medicine in Rheumatoid Arthritis: No Longer the Last Resort! HSS Journal. 2010;6(1):108-111. doi:10.1007/s11420-009-9133-8.
4. Bartlett SJ, Haaz S, Mill C, Bernatsky S, Bingham CO. Yoga in Rheumatic Diseases. Current rheumatology reports. 2013;15(12):387. doi:10.1007/s11926-013-0387-2.
5. Pradhan EK, Baumgarten M, Langenberg P, et al. Effect of Mindfulness-Based Stress Reduction in rheumatoid arthritis patients. Arthritis Rheum. 2007;57(7):1134–1142.
6. Zautra AJ, Davis MC, Reich JW, et al. Comparison of cognitive behavioral and mindfulness meditation interventions on adaptation to rheumatoid arthritis for patients with and without history of recurrent depression. J Consult Clin Psychol. 2008;76(3):408–421.
7. Haslock I, Monro R, Nagarathna R, Nagendra HR, Raghuram NV. Measuring the effects of yoga in rheumatoid arthritis. Br J Rheumatol. 1994;33(8):787–788.

8. Dash M, Telles S. Improvement in hand grip strength in normal volunteers and rheumatoid arthritis patients following yoga training. Indian J Physiol Pharmacol. 2001;45(3):355–360.

9. Badsha H, Chhabra V, Leibman C, Mofti A, Kong KO. The benefits of yoga for rheumatoid arthritis: results of a preliminary, structured 8-week program. Rheumatol Int. 2009;29(12):1417–1421.

10. Bosch PR, Traustadóttir T, Howard P, Matt KS. Functional and physiological effects of yoga in women with rheumatoid arthritis: a pilot study. Altern Ther Health Med. 2009;15(4):24–31.

11. Evans S, Moieni M, Taub R, Subramanian SK, Tsao JC, Sternlieb B, Zeltzer LK. Iyengar yoga for young adults with rheumatoid arthritis: results from a mixed-methods pilot study. J Pain Symptom Manage. 2010;39(5):904–13.

12. Telles S, Naveen KV, Gaur V, Balkrishna A. Effect of one week of yoga on function and severity in rheumatoid arthritis. BMC Res Notes. 2011;4:118.

13. Evans S, Moieni M, Lung K, et al. Impact of Iyengar yoga on quality of life in young women with rheumatoid arthritis. The Clinical journal of pain. 2013;29(11):988-997. doi:10.1097/AJP.0b013e31827da381.

Rhinitis/Sinusitis

Rhinitis is a result of inflammation of the nasal mucosa. According to the duration of nasal symptoms, rhinitis is defined as acute (resolving within 10 days) or chronic (lasting longer than 10 days). The acute form is usually associated with one or more of the following symptoms: nasal discharge, sneezing, nasal itching and congestion[1,2]. There may be other accompanying symptoms such as repeated throat clearing, headaches, facial pain, ear pain, itchy throat and palate, snoring, and sleep disturbances[3,4]. Chronic rhinitis may result in nasal obstruction. In severe cases, there may be crusting, frequent bleeding, and thick, foul-smelling, pus-filled discharge from the nose.

Rhinitis may be non-allergic or allergic. Non-allergic rhinitis is usually due to a viral infection (common cold). Allergic rhinitis is due to an allergy, usually to pollen, mold, animal dander, or dust. It is estimated that 10% to 25% of the population may develop allergic rhinitis (also known as hay fever) every year. Chronic rhinitis may affect up to 40% of the population annually[5,6].

Treatment for the common cold is usually with over the counter decongestants. Allergic rhinitis can be prevented and treated by avoiding the allergy triggers, nasal corticosteroid sprays, and antihistamines. Desensitization injections may be sometimes required. Chronic rhinitis may require decongestants. An underlying infection may be present in these patients and may require antibiotics. Rarely, a biopsy is done in resistant cases to rule out cancer.

Complimentary modalities have also been used[7]. Some yoga techniques, have also been tried[8].

Yoga and Rhinitis/Sinusitis

Nasal irrigation with saline water is used in both acute and chronic sinusitis and is in the tradition of Ayurveda/yoga[9] with beneficial results[10]. 16 ounces of lukewarm water (distilled, sterile, or previously boiled) to which one teaspoon of salt has been added, is usually used for nasal irrigation by a (nasal irrigation) device, once a day. Yoga practitioners use an irrigation pot called 'Neti'. In patients with sinusitis, nasal irrigation helps decrease symptoms, and decreases medication use[11].

Conclusion

Nasal irrigation with saline water, using 'Neti', can help by removing allergens/bacteria and discharges/crusts in these patients.

References

1. Wallace DV, Dykewicz MS, Bernstein DI, Blessing-Moore J, Cox L, Khan DA, Lang DM, Nicklas RA, Oppenheimer J, Portnoy JM, Randolph CC, Schuller D, Spector SL, Tilles SA. The diagnosis and management of rhinitis: an updated practice parameter. J Allergy Clin Immunol. 2008;122:S1–S84.
2. van Cauwenberge P, Bachert C, Passalacqua G, Bousquet J, Canonica GW, Durham SR, Fokkens WJ, Howarth PH, Lund V, Malling HJ, Mygind N, Passali D, Scadding GK, Wang DY. Consensus statement on the treatment of allergic rhinitis. European Academy of Allergology and Clinical Immunology. Allergy. 2000;55:116–134.
3. Benninger M, Farrar JR, Blaiss M, Chipps B, Ferguson B, Krouse J, Marple B, Storms W, Kaliner M. Evaluating approved medications to treat allergic rhinitis in the United States: an evidence-based review of efficacy for nasal symptoms by class. Ann Allergy Asthma Immunol. 2010;104:13–29.
4. Nathan RA. The burden of allergic rhinitis. Allergy Asthma Proc. 2007;28:3–9.
5. Tran NP, Vickery J, Blaiss MS. Management of rhinitis: allergic and non-allergic. Allergy Asthma Immunol Res. 2011;3:148–156.
6. Bousquet J, Fokkens W, Burney P, Durham SR, Bachert C, Akdis CA, Canonica GW, Dahlen SE, Zuberbier T, Bieber T, et al. Important research questions in allergy and related diseases: nonallergic rhinitis: a GA2LEN paper. Allergy. 2008;63:842–853.
7. Resnick ES, Bielory BP, Bielory L. Complementary therapy in allergic rhinitis. Curr Allergy Asthma Rep. 2008 Apr;8(2):118-25.
8. Sim MK. Treatment of disease without the use of drugs. VI. Treatment of rhinitis by a yogic process of cleaning and rubbing the nasal passage with a rubber catheter. Singapore Med J. 1981 Jun;22(3):121-3.
9. Achilles N, Mösges R. Nasal saline irrigations for the symptoms of acute and chronic rhinosinusitis. Curr Allergy Asthma Rep. 2013 Apr;13(2):229-35. doi: 10.1007/s11882-013-0339-y.
10. Adappa ND, Wei CC, Palmer JN. Nasal irrigation with or without drugs: the evidence. Curr Opin Otolaryngol Head Neck Surg. 2012 Feb;20(1):53-7. doi: 10.1097/MOO.0b013e32834dfa80.

11. Rabago D, Zgierska A, Mundt M, Barrett B, Bobula J, Maberry R. Efficacy of daily hypertonic saline nasal irrigation among patients with sinusitis: a randomized controlled trial. J Fam Pract 2002;51:1049-55.

Schizophrenia

Schizophrenia is one of the top ten causes of disability in developed countries[1]. It affects approximately one percent of the population. It usually occurs in late adolescence or early adulthood and is characterized by delusions, hallucinations, and other cognitive difficulties. Psychiatric co-morbidities are common in these patients. These include anxiety disorders[2,3] and depression[4]. Suicide is also high in patients with schizophrenia[5]. Drug abuse or dependence is often seen in this population, with 47% having a lifetime diagnosis of abuse or addiction. 34% of schizophrenia patients abuse alcohol[6]. and many are heavy smokers[7]. They also have significant medical co-morbidities that include COPD, diabetes mellitus, hypertension, hyperlipidemia and ischemic heart disease[8]. They have a lower life-span[9].

Treatment is with antipsychotics, and psychosocial interventions. Commonly used drugs include risperidone, olanzapine, quetiapine, ziprasidone, clozapine and haloperidol. These drugs are often associated with undesirable side effects and non-compliance can be high[10]. Complementary and alternative medicine modalities have also been used in these patients[11], including yoga[12].

Yoga and Schizophrenia

Visceglia and Lewis randomized, 18 clinically stable patients (12 men and 6 women) with schizophrenia (mean age=42±13.5) to an 8-week yoga therapy program and a waitlist group. Symptoms were measured using the Positive and Negative Syndrome Scale. Secondary efficacy outcomes were measured with the World Health Organization Quality of Life BREF questionnaire. In this controlled pilot study, the yoga group were found to have significant improvements in psychopathology and quality of life when compared with controls[13].

Yoga when combined with usual care in 50 patients with schizophrenia increased the level of functional recovery[14]. Physical exercise and yoga improve attention and additional cognitive domains in schizophrenia patients and the benefit lasts well past the training period[15]. However, some studies have found yoga better than regular exercise in improving the cognitive status of schizophrenia patients[16]. Cognitive function improvements in patients with schizophrenia were also reported by Bhatia and group, when yoga therapy patients were compared with usual therapy group[17]. A study of yoga in inpatients showed an improvement in associated depression in yoga patients compared to a group of physical exercise patients[18].

In a review of three randomized controlled trials, researchers found that yoga improved the quality of life in schizophrenia patients more than those exposed to physical exercise or being on the control wait list, using the World Health Organization Quality of Life questionnaire (WHOQOL-BREF)[19]. An improved quality of life in schizophrenia patients was also reported by 15 patients given yoga along with pharmacotherapy when compared to 15 patients given pharmacotherapy alone after one month[20].

In another study, a total of 43 schizophrenia patients were randomized to yoga group (n=15) or waitlist group (n=28). The study was completed by fifteen patients in the yoga group and twelve patients in the waitlist control group. The yoga group showed significant improvements in socio-occupational functioning, performance on 'tool for recognition of emotions in neuropsychiatric disorders' and plasma increase in oxytocin levels as compared with the waitlist group. This study suggested that oxytocin may play a role in the improvement in social cognition deficits in these patients[21].

Patients with schizophrenia are usually willing to do yoga and are compliant[22].

Conclusion

Studies on therapeutic yoga as a complementary treatment for schizophrenia are limited. Most studies appear to indicate benefits with yoga therapy, but this is comparable to that achieved with physical exercise. Yoga can be used in patients who are not able to do physical exercise, as an add on therapy for improving negative symptomatology and social cognition.

References

1. Murray RM, Lopez AD. Global burden disease: a comprehensive assessment of mortality and disability from diseases, injuries and risk factors in 1990 and projected to 2020. Cambridge (MA): Harvard University Press; 1996.
2. Goodwin R, Lyons JS, McNally RJ. Panic attacks in schizophrenia. Schizophr Res. 2002;58(2–3):213–220.
3. Tibbo P, Swainson J, Chue P, LeMelledo JM. Prevalence and relationship to delusions and hallucinations of anxiety disorders in schizophrenia. Depress Anxiety. 2003;17(2):65–72.
4. Siris SG. Depression in schizophrenia: perspective in the era of "Atypical" antipsychotic agents. Am J Psychiatry. 2000;157(9):1379–1389.
5. Siris SG. Suicide and schizophrenia. J Psychopharmacol. 2001;15(2):127–135.
6. Regier DA, Farmer ME, Rae DS, Locke BZ, Keith SJ, Judd LL, et al. Comorbidity of mental disorders with alcohol and other, drug abuse. Results from the Epidemiologic Catchment Area (ECA) Study. JAMA. 1990;264(19):2511–2518.
7. Sagud M, Mihaljević-Peles A, Mück-Seler D, Pivac N, Vuksan-Cusa B, Brataljenović T, Jakovljević M. Smoking and schizophrenia. Psychiatr Danub. 2009 Sep;21(3):371-5.
8. Carney CP, Jones L, Woolson RF. Medical Comorbidity in Women and Men with Schizophrenia: A Population-Based Controlled Study. Journal of General Internal Medicine. 2006;21(11):1133-1137. doi:10.1111/j.1525-1497.2006.00563.x.
9. Thornicroft G. Physical health disparities and mental illness: the scandal of premature mortality. Br J Psychiatry. 2011;199:441–442.
10. de Araújo AA1, de Araújo Dantas D, do Nascimento GG et al. Quality of life in patients with schizophrenia: the impact of socio-economic factors and adverse effects of atypical antipsychotics drugs. Psychiatr Q. 2014 Sep;85(3):357-67. doi: 10.1007/s11126-014-9290-x.
11. Babić D, Babić R. Complementary and alternative medicine in the treatment of schizophrenia. Psychiatr Danub. 2009 Sep;21(3):376-81.
12. Broderick J, Vancampfort D. Yoga as part of a package of care versus standard care for schizophrenia. Cochrane Database Syst Rev. 2017 Sep 29;9:CD012145. doi: 10.1002/14651858.CD012145.pub2.
13. Visceglia E, Lewis S. Yoga therapy as an adjunctive treatment for schizophrenia: a randomized, controlled pilot study. J Altern Complement Med. 2011 Jul;17(7):601-7. doi: 10.1089/acm.2010.0075.
14. Kavak F, Ekinci M. The Effect of Yoga on Functional Recovery Level in Schizophrenic Patients. Arch Psychiatr Nurs. 2016 Dec;30(6):761-767. doi: 10.1016/j.apnu.2016.07.010. Epub 2016 Jul 30.
15. Bhatia T, Mazumdar S, Wood J3, He F, Gur RE, Gur RC, Nimgaonkar VL, Deshpande SN. A randomised controlled trial of adjunctive yoga and adjunctive physical exercise training for cognitive dysfunction in

schizophrenia. Acta Neuropsychiatr. 2017 Apr;29(2):102-114. doi: 10.1017/neu.2016.42. Epub 2016 Aug 12.

16. Varambally S, Gangadhar BN, Thirthalli J, et al. Therapeutic efficacy of add-on yogasana intervention in stabilized outpatient schizophrenia: Randomized controlled comparison with exercise and waitlist. Indian Journal of Psychiatry. 2012;54(3):227-232. doi:10.4103/0019-5545.102414.

17. Bhatia T, Agarwal A, Shah G, et al. Adjunctive cognitive remediation for schizophrenia using yoga: an open, non-randomized trial. Acta neuropsychiatrica: officieel wetenschappelijk orgaan van het IGBP (Interdisciplinair Genootschap voor Biologische Psychiatrie). 2012;24(2):91-100. doi:10.1111/j.1601-5215.2011.00587.x.

18. Manjunath RB. Bangalore: Psychiatry, National Institute of Mental Health and Neurosciences; 2009. Efficacy of yoga therapy as an add-on treatment for in-patients and out-patients with functional psychotic disorder [Dissertation].

19. Vancampfort D, Vansteelandt K, Scheewe T, Probst M, Knapen J, De Herdt A, De Hert M. Yoga in schizophrenia: a systematic review of randomised controlled trials. Acta Psychiatr Scand. 2012 Jul;126(1):12-20. doi: 10.1111/j.1600-0447.2012.01865.x. Epub 2012 Apr 6.

20. Paikkatt B, Singh AR, Singh PK, Jahan M, Ranjan JK. Efficacy of Yoga therapy for the management of psychopathology of patients having chronic schizophrenia. Indian Journal of Psychiatry. 2015;57(4):355-360. doi:10.4103/0019-5545.171837.

21. Jayaram N, Varambally S, Behere RV, et al. Effect of yoga therapy on plasma oxytocin and facial emotion recognition deficits in patients of schizophrenia. Indian Journal of Psychiatry. 2013;55(Suppl 3): S409-S413. doi:10.4103/0019-5545.116318.

22. Govindaraj R, Varambally S, Gangadhar BN. Yoga for schizophrenia: Patients' perspective. International Journal of Yoga. 2015;8(2):139-141. doi:10.4103/0973-6131.154077.

Scoliosis

Idiopathic scoliosis is a complex deformity of the spine. It is characterized by a lateral deviation of more than 10 degree along with axial rotation[1-5]. The exact etiology is unknown. Genetic factors appear to play a major role in its pathogenesis[6]. Its prevalence is approximately 2%-4% in adolescents[7], and girls are more likely to progress to a severe form[8,9].

Several classifications exist. In 1954 James classified scoliosis according to the onset: infantile, from birth to 2 years; juvenile from 3 to 9 years, and adolescent from 10 years to maturity[10]. Another classification is based on the etiology - congenital, neuromuscular, or idiopathic. Adolescent idiopathic scoliosis (85% of the cases) is the most common form[11]. Physical examination is combined with Adam's forward bend test and a scoliometer measurement for diagnosis[12]. The Cobb angle (measurement of the degree of scoliosis on the posteroanterior radiograph) helps treatment decisions. Curves less than 10 to 15 degrees usually require no active treatment, while curves greater than 45 degrees in adolescents and greater than 50 degrees in adults, may require rod placement and bone grafting[13]. Moderate curves between 25 and 45 degrees in patients lacking skeletal maturity may require bracing[14]. Braces are usually a thoracolumbar-sacral orthosis or a cervico-thoracolumbar-sacral orthosis. Braces are used from eight to 24 hours each day, depending on the style of brace chosen. Other treatment modalities such as physical therapy, chiropractic care, and electrical stimulation have been used but without good results[15].

Scoliosis may not cause any problems or can result in visible deformity and emotional distress. Rarely respiratory impairment may arise from rib deformity[16,17].

Yoga and Scoliosis

Monroe reported a case of a 46-year-old woman with idiopathic scoliosis who was given conservative treatment including Iyengar Yoga with subjective improvement[18].

In a study evaluating the side plank pose, Fishman and associates recruited twenty-five patients with idiopathic or degenerative scoliosis and primary curves measuring 6 to 120 degrees by the Cobb method. They were taught to perform the side plank pose with convexity downward for a minimum of 10 to 20 seconds and advised to maintain the posture once daily for as long as possible on that one side only. Pre- and post-yoga Cobb measurements were compared. Patients performing the side plank pose showed a significant improvement in the Cobb angle of the primary scoliotic curve of 32.0%[19].

Conclusion

The side plank pose may have value in the treatment of some cases of mild scoliosis.

References

1. Asher MA, Burton DC. A concept of idiopathic scoliosis deformities as imperfect torsion(s) Clin Orthop Relat Res. 1999;364:11–25.
2. Reamy BV, Slakey JB. Adolescent idiopathic scoliosis: review and current concepts. Am Fam Physician. 2001;64(1):111–116.
3. Smith JR, Sciubba DM, Samdani AF. Scoliosis: a straightforward approach to diagnosis and management. JAAPA. 2008;21(11):40–45.
4. Charles YP, Dimeglio A, Marcoul M, Bourgin JF, Marcoul A, Bozonnat MC. Influence of idiopathic scoliosis on three-dimensional thoracic growth. Spine (Phila Pa 1976) 2008;33:1209–1218. doi: 10.1097/BRS.0b013e3181715272.
5. Stokes IA. Three-dimensional terminology of spinal deformity. A report presented to the scoliosis research society by the scoliosis research society working group on 3-D terminology of spinal deformity. Spine (Phila Pa 1976) 1994;19:236–248. doi: 10.1097/00007632-199401001-00020.
6. Miller NH. Genetics of familial idiopathic scoliosis. Clin Orthop Relat Res. 2007;462:6–10. ; Ogilvie J. Adolescent idiopathic scoliosis and genetic testing. Curr Opin Pediatr. 2010;22(1):67–70.
7. Smith JR, Sciubba DM, Samdani AF. Scoliosis: a straightforward approach to diagnosis and management. JAAPA. 2008;21(11):40–45.
8. O'Connor F. Pediatric Orthopedics for the Family Physician. Infant, Child & Adolescent Medicine. AAFP CME Program. 2007.
9. Weiss HR. Adolescent idiopathic scoliosis (AIS) – an indication for surgery? A systematic review of the literature. Disabil Rehabil. 2008;30(10):799–807.
10. James JI. Idiopathic scoliosis; the prognosis, diagnosis, and operative indications related to curve patterns and the age at onset. J Bone Joint Surg Br. 1954;36-B:36–49.

11. Neinstein LS, Chorley JN. Scoliosis and kyphosis. Adolescent Health Care: A Practical Guide. 4th ed. Philadelphia, Pa.: Lippincott Williams & Wilkins; 2002:345–355.
12. Horne JP, Flannery R, Usman S. Adolescent idiopathic scoliosis: diagnosis and management. Am Fam Physician. 2014 Feb 1;89(3):193-8.
13. Bridwell KH. Surgical treatment of idiopathic adolescent scoliosis. Spine (Phila Pa 1976) 1999;24:2607–2616. doi: 10.1097/00007632-199912150-00008.
14. Nachemson AL, Peterson LE. Effectiveness of treatment with a brace in girls who have adolescent idiopathic scoliosis. A prospective, controlled study based on data from the brace study of the scoliosis research society. J Bone Joint Surg Am. 1995;77:815–822.
15. Reamy BV, Slakey JB. Adolescent idiopathic scoliosis: review and current concepts. Am Fam Physician. 2001;64(1):111–116.
16. Weiss HR. Adolescent idiopathic scoliosis (AIS) – an indication for surgery? A systematic review of the literature. Disabil Rehabil. 2008;30(10):799–807.
17. Glassman SD, Carreon LY, Shaffrey CI, et al. The costs and benefits of nonoperative management for adult scoliosis. Spine (Phila Pa 1976). 2010;35(5):578–582.
18. Marcia Monroe. Scoliosis. 2010; 5(Suppl 1): O24. Published online 2010 Sep 10.
19. Loren M. Fishman, Erik J. Groessl, Karen J. Sherman. Serial Case Reporting Yoga for Idiopathic and Degenerative Scoliosis. Glob Adv Health Med. 2014 Sep; 3(5): 16–21.

Smoking Cessation

Smoking involves burning the dried leaves of the tobacco plant, rolled into a cigarette, and breathing in the resulting smoke. This activity dates to about 5000 BCE. Tobacco smoke is a complex mixture of over 5,000 identified chemicals, many of them toxic and carcinogenic. The main active compound is an alkaloid, called nicotine. Nicotine is a stimulant and highly addictive. Smoking is associated with a plethora of deleterious health conditions, including cardiovascular disease, COPD, diabetes mellitus, poor dental health, rheumatoid arthritis and cataracts. It also affects men's fertility and can cause significant problems during pregnancy. It is the number one preventable cause of death worldwide.

Approximately 15% of the American adult population smokes[1]. Smoking is responsible for more than 480,000 deaths each year in the United States. It is responsible for more deaths each year than the combined number of deaths from, human immunodeficiency virus, illegal drug use. alcohol use, motor vehicle injuries and firearm-related incidents[2].

Smoking is also a major and independent risk factor for cardiovascular disease, including atherosclerotic vascular disease, hypertension, myocardial infarction, unstable angina, sudden cardiac death, and stroke[3,4]. Smoking increases the risk of coronary heart disease and stroke by 2 to 4 times. According to an epidemiological study >1 in 10 cardiovascular deaths, which make up 54% of all deaths worldwide, are related to smoking[5].

Smoking increases the risk of lung cancer and many other cancers, including cancer of the bladder, blood (acute myeloid leukemia), cervix, colon and rectum, esophagus, kidney and ureter, larynx, liver, oropharynx, pancreas, stomach, trachea, bronchus, and lung. Smoking is responsible for about 90% of all lung cancer deaths[6].

Smoking risks diminish after smoking cessation. The risk for heart attacks declines sharply after one year, while the risk of stroke is reduced to that of a non-smoker in 2-5 years[7]. The risk for lung cancer drops by half after ten years, while the risk for cancers of the mouth, throat, esophagus, and bladder drop by half within 5 years[7]. Women, compared to men, may be more susceptible to smoking-related morbidity and mortality[8].

Several pharmacologic agents are available for smoking cessation and include, nicotine replacement products available as transdermal patch, gum, nasal spray, inhaler and lozenges[9]. Non-nicotine replacement drugs include bupropion and varenicline[10]. Nortriptyline and clonidine have also found to be effective.

Treatment is difficult due to common barriers such as addiction[11], fear of weight gain[12] and depression[13] Most smokers find it difficult to quit smoking[14]. Complementary and alternative techniques, including yoga, are commonly used by smokers to quit smoking[15,16].

Yoga and Smoking Cessation

Yoga has been investigated in the treatment of smoking addiction[17,18]. Stress and negative mood is a strong barrier to smoking cessation[19,20]. Yoga helps reduce stress and improve mood and well-being[21] and can also help with weight loss[22]. These benefits of yoga help in smoking cessation.

In an 8-week study, fifty-five women who had received an 8-week group-based cognitive behavioral therapy for smoking cessation, were randomized to a twice-weekly program of Vinyasa yoga or a control group attending a general health and wellness program. At the end of the treatment, researchers found that yoga practitioners had a higher abstinence rate than controls, and this remained higher at the end of six months. The yoga group also showed reduced anxiety and improvements in perceived health and well-being when compared with controls[23]. In a review of four studies, Todd and associates found that the practice of yoga helped smokers quit. The yoga practitioners had increased desire and motivation to quit smoking. They had fewer urges to smoke and demonstrated reduced temptations to smoke[24].

Mindfulness meditation has also shown potential in smoking cessation. In a study of 88 nicotine-dependent adults (smoking an average of 20 cigarettes/day), were randomly assigned to receive mindfulness training or the American Lung Association's (ALA) freedom from smoking treatment. Both treatments were delivered twice weekly over 4 weeks (eight sessions total) in a group format, for 4 weeks. Mindfulness training participants were able to reduce cigarette use much more when compared to those randomized to the ALA freedom from smoking group[25]. In a review of the literature Carim-Todd and associates also reported that meditation-based therapies do help in smoking cessation[26].

Yogic breathing has also shown to reduce the craving for cigarettes[27]. In a review of 19 randomized controlled trials, Klinsophon and group concluded that yoga when combined with coginitive-behavioral therapy had a positive effect on smoking cessation[28].

In general, published data suggests that yoga as an adjunct therapy is beneficial and acceptable in patients who want to quit smoking[29]. Both men and women are open to this complimentary modality[30-31].

Conclusion

Yoga modalities may help in smoking cessation.

References

1. Jamal A, Phillips E, Gentzke AS, et al. Current Cigarette Smoking Among Adults — United States, 2016. MMWR Morb Mortal Wkly Rep 2018;67:53–59. DOI: http://dx.doi.org/10.15585/mmwr.mm6702a1.
2. Mokdad AH, Marks JS, Stroup DF, Gerberding JL. Actual Causes of Death in the United States. JAMA: Journal of the American Medical Association 2004;291(10):1238–45.
3. Ambrose JA, Barua RS. The pathophysiology of cigarette smoking and cardiovascular disease: an update. J Am Coll Cardiol 43: 1731–1737, 2004.
4. White WB. Smoking-related morbidity and mortality in the cardiovascular setting. Prev Cardiol 10, Suppl 2: 1–4, 2007.
5. Ezzati M, Henley SJ, Thun MJ, Lopez AD. Role of smoking in global and regional cardiovascular mortality. Circulation 112: 489–497, 2005.
6. U.S. Department of Health and Human Services.The Health Consequences of Smoking—50 Years of Progress: A Report of the Surgeon General. Atlanta: U.S. Department of Health and Human Services, Centers for Disease Control and Prevention, National Center for Chronic Disease Prevention and Health Promotion, Office on Smoking and Health, 2014.

7. U.S. Department of Health and Human Services. How Tobacco Smoke Causes Disease: What It Means to You. Atlanta: U.S. Department of Health and Human Services, Centers for Disease Control and Prevention, National Center for Chronic Disease Prevention and Health Promotion, Office on Smoking and Health, 2010.
8. Allen AM, Oncken C, Hatsukami D. Women and Smoking: The Effect of Gender on the Epidemiology, Health Effects, and Cessation of Smoking. Current addiction reports. 2014;1(1):53-60. doi:10.1007/s40429-013-0003-6.
9. Fiore MC, Jaén CR, Baker TB, et al. Treating Tobacco Use and Dependence: 2008 Update—Clinical Practice Guidelines. Rockville (MD): U.S. Department of Health and Human Services, Public Health Service, Agency for Healthcare Research and Quality, 2008.
10. Tønnesen P, Tonstad S, Hjalmarson A, Lebargy F, Van Spiegel PI, Hider A, et al. A multicentre, randomized, double-blind, placebo-controlled, 1-year study of bupropion SR for smoking cessation. J Intern Med. 2003;254:184–92.
11. Kenkel D, Chen L. Consumer information and tobacco use. In: Jha P, Chaloupka FJ, editors. Tobacco Control in Developing Countries. Oxford: Oxford University Press; 2000. pp. 77–214.
12. Hajek P, Jackson P, Belcher M. Long-term use of nicotine chewing gum. Occurrence, determinants and effect on weight gain. JAMA. 1988;260:1593–6.
13. Glassman AH. Cigarette smoking: Implications for psychiatric illness. Am J Psychiatry. 1993;150:546–53.
14. Hughes JR. Peters EN. Naud S. Relapse to smoking after 1 year of abstinence: a meta-analysis. Addict Behav. 2008;33:1516–1520.
15. Carim-Todd L, Mitchell SH, Oken BS. Mind-body practices: an alternative, drug-free treatment for smoking cessation? A systematic review of the literature. Drug and alcohol dependence. 2013;132(3):399-410. doi:10.1016/j.drugalcdep.2013.04.014.
16. Dai CL, Sharma M. Between inhale and exhale: yoga as an intervention in smoking cessation. J Evid Based Complementary Altern Med. 2014 Apr;19(2):144-9.
17. McIver S, O'Halloran P, McGartland M. The impact of Hatha yoga on smoking behavior. Altern Ther Health Med. 2004 Mar-Apr;10(2):22-3.
18. Andrea Elibero, M.A. Kate Janse Van Rensburg, Ph.D David J. Drobes, Ph.D. Acute Effects of Aerobic Exercise and Hatha Yoga on Craving to Smoke. Nicotine & Tobacco Research, Volume 13, Issue 11, 1 November 2011, Pages 1140–1148.
19. Zeger SL. Liang KY. Feedback models for discrete and continuous time series. Statistica Sinica. 1991;1:51–64.
20. Kassel JD. Stroud LR. Paronis CA. Smoking, stress, and negative affect: correlation, causation, and context across stages of smoking. Psychol Bull. 2003;129:270–304.
21. Mishra RS. Fundamentals of Yoga: A Handbook of Theory, Practice and Applications. New York: Harmony Books; 1987.

22. Bera TK, Rajapurkar MV. Body composition, cardiovascular endurance and anaerobic power of yogic practitioner. Indian J Physiol Pharmacol. 1993;37:225–8.
23. Bock BC, Fava JL, Gaskins R, et al. Yoga as a Complementary Treatment for Smoking Cessation in Women. Journal of Women's Health. 2012;21(2):240-248. doi:10.1089/jwh.2011.2963.
24. L Carim Todd, S Mitchell, B Oken. Does yoga improve smoking cessation outcomes? A systematic review of the literature. BMC Complement Altern Med. 2012; 12(Suppl 1): P389. Published online 2012 Jun 12.
25. Brewer JA, Mallik S, Babuscio TA, Nich C, Johnson HE, Deleone CM, Minnix-Cotton CA, Byrne SA, Kober H, Weinstein AJ, Carroll KM, Rounsaville BJ. Mindfulness training for smoking cessation: results from a randomized controlled trial. Drug Alcohol Depend. 2011;119:72–80.
26. Carim-Todd L, Mitchell SH, Oken BS. Mind-body practices: an alternative, drug-free treatment for smoking cessation? A systematic review of the literature. Drug and alcohol dependence. 2013;132(3):399-410. doi:10.1016/j.drugalcdep.2013.04.014.
27. Shahab L, Sarkar BK, West R. The acute effects of yogic breathing exercises on craving and withdrawal symptoms in abstaining smokers. Psychopharmacology (Berl). 2013 Feb;225(4):875-82.
28. Klinsophon T, Thaveeratitham P, Sitthipornvorakul E, Janwantanakul P. Effect of exercise type on smoking cessation: a meta-analysis of randomized controlled trials. BMC Research Notes. 2017;10:442. doi:10.1186/s13104-017-2762-y.
29. Rosen RK, Thind H, Jennings E, Guthrie KM, Williams DM, Bock BC. "Smoking Does Not Go with Yoga:" A Qualitative Study of Women's Phenomenological Perceptions During Yoga and Smoking Cessation. Int J Yoga Therap. 2016 Jan;26(1):33-41.
30. Thind H, Jennings E, Fava JL, et al. Differences between Men and Women Enrolling in Smoking Cessation Programs Using Yoga as a Complementary Therapy. Journal of yoga & physical therapy. 2016;6(3):245. doi:10.4172/2157-7595.1000245.
31. Bock BC, Thind H, Dunsiger S, Fava JL, Jennings E, Becker BM, Marcus BH, Rosen RK, Sillice MA. Who Enrolls in a Quit Smoking Program with Yoga Therapy? Am J Health Behav. 2017 Nov 1;41(6):740-749.

Urinary Incontinence

Urinary incontinence (UI) is associated with significant morbidity. It is estimated that approximately 10 million patients in the U.S. have UI. It is more common in women, at age 80 or under. UI is often associated with hypertension and depression[1,2]. Women with UI also experience social isolation, physical inactivity, falls and fractures and premature nursing home placement[3-6]. They also experience a decreased quality of life[7]. Symptoms may include urine urgency, leakage of urine with coughing or sneezing and in men, dribbling[8,9]. Urodynamic studies are helpful in the diagnostic process[10].

Treatment may include anti-cholinergic medications and behavioral treatments[11,12].

Yoga and Urinary Incontinence

In a pilot randomized trial of ten ambulatory women aged 40 years and older with stress, urgency, or mixed-type incontinence, yoga therapy program was given as twice weekly group classes and once weekly home practice. The waitlist control group had nine women. After 6 weeks, total incontinence frequency decreased by 66% in the yoga therapy group versus 13% in the control group (P=0.049). Participants in the yoga therapy group also reported an average of 85% decrease in stress incontinence frequency compared to a 25% increase in controls[13].

Conclusion

Yoga may help improve urinary incontinence. More studies are needed.

References

1. Minassian VA, Stewart WF, Wood GC. Urinary incontinence in women: Variation in prevalence estimates and risk factors. Obstet Gynecol. 2008;111(2 Part 1):324–331.
2. Markland AD, Goode PS, Redden DT, et al. Prevalence of urinary incontinence in men: Results from the national health and nutrition examination survey. J Urol. 2010;84(3):1022–1027.
3. Thom DH, Haan MN, Van Den Eeden SK. Medically recognized urinary incontinence and risks of hospitalization, nursing home admission and mortality. Age Ageing. 1997 Sep;26(5):367–374.

4. Fultz NH, Fisher GG, Jenkins KR. Does urinary incontinence affect middle-aged and older women's time use and activity patterns? Obstet Gynecol. 2004 Dec;104(6):1327–1334.

5. Brown JS, Vittinghoff E, Wyman JF, et al. Urinary incontinence: does it increase risk for falls and fractures? Study of Osteoporotic Fractures Research Group. J Am Geriatr Soc. 2000 Jul;48(7):721–725.

6. Lawhorne LW, Ouslander JG, Parmelee PA, et al. Urinary incontinence: A neglected geriatric syndrome in nursing facilities. J Am Med Dir Assoc. 2008;9(1):29–35.

7. Avery JC, Stocks NP, Duggan P, et al. Identifying the quality of life effects of urinary incontinence with depression in an Australian population. BMC Urology. 2013;13:11. doi:10.1186/1471-2490-13-11.

8. Tannenbaum C, Perrin L, DuBeau C, et al. Diagnosis and management of urinary incontinence in the older patient. Arch Phys Med Rehabil. 2001;82:134–138.

9. Scientific Committee of the First International Consultation on Incontinence Assessment and treatment of urinary incontinence. Lancet. 2000;355:2153–2158.

10. Housley SL, Harding C, Pickard R. Urodynamic assessment of urinary incontinence. Indian Journal of Urology□: IJU□: Journal of the Urological Society of India. 2010;26(2):215-220. doi:10.4103/0970-1591.65392.

11. Shamliyan T, Wyman J, Kane RL. Nonsurgical Treatments for Urinary Incontinence in Adult Women: Diagnosis and Comparative Effectiveness. Rockville MD: 2012.

12. Wyman JF, Fantl JA, McClish DK, et al. Comparative efficacy of behavioral interventions in the management of female urinary incontinence. Continence Program for Women Research Group. Am J Obstet Gynecol. 1998 Oct;179(4):999–1007.

13. Huang AJ, Jenny HE, Chesney MA, Schembri M, Subak LL. A Group-Based Yoga Therapy Intervention for Urinary Incontinence in Women: A Pilot Randomized Trial. Female pelvic medicine & reconstructive surgery. 2014;20(3):147-154. doi:10.1097/SPV.0000000000000072.

Miscellaneous Conditions

Musculo-skeletal Disorders

Musculoskeletal pain is common in dentists, with 34.5% reporting this symptom. Yoga practice reduced this percentage to 10.5%, compared to 21.7% in control dentists with other physical activity and 45.6% in dentists with no physical activity.

Koneru S, Tanikonda R. Role of yoga and physical activity in work-related musculoskeletal disorders among dentists. Journal of International Society of Preventive & Community Dentistry. 2015;5(3):199-204. doi:10.4103/2231-0762.159957.

Neurodegenerative Disorders

A case report on the successful use of yoga (10 months) as therapy for a rare neurological disorder, adrenomyeloneuropathy. The patient experienced improvements in agility, balance, and walking, and overall quality of life.

Charlene Marie Muhammad, Steffany Haaz Moonaz. Yoga as Therapy for Neurodegenerative Disorders: A Case Report of Therapeutic Yoga for Adrenomyeloneuropathy. Integr Med (Encinitas) 2014 Jun; 13(3): 33–39.

Pancreatitis

In a randomized study, patients in the yoga group (biweekly yoga for 12 weeks) reported significant improvements in overall quality of life, symptoms of stress, mood changes, alcohol dependence and appetite when compared to the control group.

Surinder Sareen, Vinita Kumari, Karaminder Singh Gajebasia, Nimanpreet Kaur Gajebasia. Yoga: A tool for improving the quality of life in chronic pancreatitis. World J Gastroenterol. 2007 Jan 21; 13(3): 391–397.

Parkinson's Disease

In a randomized controlled pilot study, thirteen people with stage 1-2 Parkinson's disease were assigned a yoga group (n = 8) or a control group (n = 5). The yoga group participated in twice-weekly yoga sessions for 12 weeks. At the end of the study, significant improvement in Unified Parkinson's Disease Rating Scale scores, diastolic blood pressure, and average forced vital capacity was noted in the yoga group. The yoga group also had improvements in depression scores, body weight, and forced expiratory volume. They also reported immediate tremor reduction.

Neena K Sharma, Kristin Robbins, Kathleen Wagner, Yvonne M Colgrove. A randomized controlled pilot study of the therapeutic effects of yoga in people with Parkinson's disease. Int J Yoga. 2015 Jan-Jun; 8(1): 74–79. doi: 10.4103/0973-6131.146070.

Periodontitis

A cross-sectional pilot study recruited 70 subjects (ages 35-60 years) with chronic periodontitis. They were divided into group I (with stress), group II (without stress), and group III (practicing yoga). Psychological evaluation was carried out using Hamilton Anxiety Rating Scale (HAM-A) and Zung Self-rating Depression Scale (ZSDS). Periodontal parameters like plaque index, probing pocket depth, and clinical attachment level at 5–8 mm and >8 mm were measured and recorded. Serum cortisol levels were also measured. Cross-sectional observation done revealed that the yoga group had low serum cortisol levels, HAM-A scale and ZSDS scores, and better periodontal health.

Kishore Kumar Katuri, Ankineedu Babu Dasari, Sruthi Kurapati, Narayana Rao Vinnakota, Appaiah Chowdary Bollepalli, Ravindranath Dhulipalla. Association of yoga practice and serum cortisol levels in chronic periodontitis patients with stress-related anxiety and depression. J Int Soc Prev Community Dent. 2016 Jan-Feb; 6(1): 7–14. doi: 10.4103/2231-0762.175404.

Pleural Effusion

Ten patients with pleural effusion practiced alternate nostril breathing for 20 days after aspiration of fluid. Researchers measured several lung parameters, at regular intervals. They reported that breathing exercises resulted in a quicker re-expansion of the lungs.

Prakasamma M, Bhaduri A. A study of yoga as a nursing intervention in the care of patients with pleural effusion. J Adv. Nurs. 1984 Mar;9(2):127-33.

Post-Operative Recovery

Researchers had patients after upper abdominal surgery do lung exercises for 10 minutes, twice daily, for five post-operative days. (using a new device,'Pink City Lung Exerciser'). They reported a significantly low incidence of pulmonary complications and better recovery of pulmonary functions in patients doing pranayama exercises.

Tyagi I; Sharma UD; Bajaj P; Husain T; Gupta S; Lamba PS; Khan A. Evaluation of pink city lung exerciser for prevention of pulmonary complications following upper abdominal surgery. Indian Journal of Anaesthesia. 1991 Dec; 39(6): 198-203.

Psoriasis

Mindfulness meditation-based stress reduction intervention can increase the rate of resolution of psoriatic lesions in patients with psoriasis.

Bernhard, J., Kristeller, J. and Kabat-Zinn, J. Effectiveness of relaxation and visualization techniques as a adjunct to phototherapy and photochemotherapy of psoriasis. J. Am. Acad. Dermatol. (1988) 19:572-73.

Psychosis

A total of 140 female patients were recruited, and 124 received the allocated intervention in a randomized controlled study of 12 weeks of yoga or aerobic exercise compared with a waitlist group.

Benefits were seen in both exercise groups. However, the yoga group showed additional benefits in verbal acquisition and attention, when compared to the aerobic exercise group.

Jingxia Lin, Sherry KW Chan, Edwin HM Lee, Wing Chung Chang, Michael Tse, Wayne Weizhong Su, Pak Sham, Christy LM Hui, Glen Joe, Cecilia LW Chan, P L Khong, Kwok Fai So, William G Honer, Eric YH Chen. Aerobic exercise and yoga improve neurocognitive function in women with early psychosis. NPJ Schizophr. 2015; 1(0): 15047.

Tuberculosis

In a prospective, randomized trial 73 tuberculosis patients were alternately allocated, to yoga (n = 36) or breath awareness (n = 37) groups. The practice was for 6 hours per week, each session being 60 min. At the end of 2 months, the yoga group showed a significant reduction in symptom scores, and an increase in weight, forced vital capacity and forced expiratory volume. Sputum conversion and an improvement in the radiographic picture was noted to be more in the yoga group.

Visweswaraiah NK, Telles S. Randomized trial of yoga as a complementary therapy for pulmonary tuberculosis. Respirology. 2004 Mar;9(1):96-101.

RESOURCES

Books

- Principles and Practice of Yoga in Health Care. Sat Bir Khalsa, Lorenzo Cohen, Timothy McCall, Shirley Telles. Handspring Publishing.
- Yoga as Medicine: The Yogic Prescription for Health and Healing. Timothy Mccall. Bantam.
- Medical Therapeutic Yoga. Ginger Garner. Handspring Publishing.

Professional Yoga Associations

- iayt.org (International Association of Yoga Therapists)
- yogaalliance.org (Yoga Alliance)

Professional Medical Associations

- ADHD: add.org (Attention Deficit Disorder Association)
- Alcohol Use Disorder: niaaa.org (National Institute on Alcohol Abuse and Alcoholism)
- Alzheimer's Disease: alz.org (Alzheimer's Association)
- Anxiety: adaa.org (Anxiety and Depression Association of America); psychiatry.org (American Psychiatry Association)
- Asthma: aaaai.org (American Association of Allergy, Asthma and Immunology); aafa.org (Asthma and Allergy Foundation of America)
- Autism: autism-society.org (Autism Society of America)

- Back Pain: americanpainsociety.org (American Pain Society)
- Cancer: cancer.gov (National Cancer Institute)
- Cardiac Rehabilitation: heart.org (American Heart Association)
- Carpel Tunnel: aanem.org (American Association for Neuromuscular and Electrodiagnostic Medicine)
- Chronic Fatigue Syndrome: acfsme.org (International Association for Chronic Fatigue Syndrome/Myalgic Encephalomyelitis); ncf-net.org (The National CFIDS Foundation)
- Chronic Kidney Disease: kidney.org (National Kidney Foundation)
- COPD: copdfoundation.org (COPD Foundation); lung.org (American Lung Association)
- Coronary Artery Disease: Heart.org (American Heart Association)
- CHF: hfsa.org (Heart Failure Society of America)
- Depression: adaa.org (Anxiety and Depression Association of America); psychiatry.org (American Psychiatry Association)
- Diabetes Mellitus: diabetes.org (American Diabetes Association)
- Drug addiction/withdrawal: asam.org (American Society of Addiction Medicine); drugabuse.gov (National Institute on Drug Abuse)
- Eating disorders: aedweb.org (Academy of Eating Disorders); apa.org (American Psychological Association); nationaleatingdisorders.org (National Eating Disorders Association); anad.org (National Association of Anorexia Nervosa and Associated Disorders)
- Epilepsy: epilepsy.org (Epilepsy Foundation)
- Fibromyalgia: fmaware.org (National Fibromyalgia Association)
- Hypertension: heart.org (American Heart Association); ish-world.com (International Society of Hypertension)

- HIV/AIDS: hivma.org (HIV Medicine Association); iasociety.org (International AIDS Society); aahivm.org (American Academy of HIV Medicine)
- Infertility: resolve.org (National Infertility Association); americanpregnancy.org (American Pregnancy Association)
- Insomnia: aasm.org (American Academy of Sleep Medicine)
- Irritable Bowel Syndrome: gastro.org (American Gastroenterological Association); ibsgroup.org (Irritable Bowel Syndrome Association)
- Menopausal Disorders: menopause.org (North American Menopause Society); imsociety.org (International Menopause Society)
- Menstrual Disorders: acog.org (American College of Obstetricians and Gynecologists); aap.org (American Academy of Pediatrics)
- Metabolic Syndrome: heart.org (American Heart Association)
- Migraine: americanmigrainefoundation.org (American Migraine Foundation); headaches.org (National Headache Foundation);
- Multiple Sclerosis: nationalmssociety.org (National Multiple Sclerosis Society); mymsaa.org (Multiple Sclerosis Association of America)
- Musculo-skeletal disorders: nih.gov (National Institute of Arthritis and Musculoskeletal and Skin Diseases)
- Neurodegenerative Disorders: indd.org (Institute for Neurodegenerative Disorders)
- Obesity: obesity.org (The Obesity Society); heart.org (American Heart Association)
- Obsessive compulsive disorder: adaa.org (Anxiety and Depression Association of America); iocdf.org (International OCD Foundation)
- Osteoarthritis: arthritis.org (Arthritis Foundation)
- Osteoporosis: nof.org (National Osteoporosis Foundation); iofbonehealth.org (International Osteoporosis Foundation)

- Pancreatitis: American-pancreatic-association.org (American Pancreatic Association); gastro.org (American Gastroenterological Association)
- Parkinson's Disease: apdaparkinson.org (American Parkinson Disease Association); Parkinson.org (Parkinson's Foundation)
- Periodontitis: perio.org (American Academy of Periodontology)
- Psychosis: psychiatry.org (American Psychiatry Association)
- Pleural Effusion: lung.org (American Lung Association); thoracic.org (American Thoracic Society)
- Polycystic Ovaries: pcosaa.org (Polycystic Ovarian Syndrome Awareness Association)
- Post-op Recovery: aserhq.org (American Society for Enhanced Recovery)
- Post stroke rehabilitation: strokeassociation.org (American Stroke Association); stroke.org (National Stroke Association)
- Pregnancy/Perinatal Disorders: americanpregnancy.org (American Pregnancy Association); acog.org (American College of Obstetricians and Gynecologists)
- Psoriasis: psoriasis.org (National Psoriasis Foundation)
- PTSD: adaa.org (Anxiety and Depression Association of America); ptsd.va.gov (US Department of Veteran Affairs/National Center for PTSD); psychiatry.org (American Psychiatry Association)
- Restless leg syndrome: rls.org (Restless Legs Syndrome Foundation); aanem.org (American Association of Neuromuscular & Electrodiagnostic Medicine); sleepfoundation.org (National Sleep Foundation)
- Rheumatoid arthritis: arthritis.org (Arthritis Foundation)
- Rhinitis/Sinusitis: aafa.org (Asthma and Allergy Foundation of America); entnet.org (American Academy of Otolaryngology–Head and Neck Surgery)
- Schizophrenia: nami.org (National Alliance on Mental Illness); psychiatry.org (American Psychiatry Association);

sardaa.org (Schizophrenia and Related Disorders Alliance of America)

- Scoliosis: scoliosis.org (National Scoliosis Foundation); srs.org (Scoliosis Research Society)
- Smoking cessation: lung.org (American Lung Association); cancer.org (American Cancer Society); thoracic.org (American Thoracic Society); heart.org (American Heart Association)
- Tuberculosis: lung.org (American Lung Association)
- Urinary Incontinence: urologyhealth.org (Urology Care Foundation)

INDEX

C

D

E

ejection fraction[22] · 11
epilepsy · 123, 124, 125, 238
epinephrine · 12
exercise · 10, 15, 17, 28, 30, 37, 40, 45, 52, 53, 57, 58, 62, 63, 65, 68, 69, 70, 78, 82, 87, 91, 93, 94, 95, 96, 97, 103, 104, 130, 133, 144, 147, 149, 157, 158, 159, 160, 162, 164, 170, 173, 174, 175, 176, 178, 179, 181, 191, 196, 198, 211, 212, 219, 220, 221, 222, 229, 230, 235, 236

F

fatigue · 34, 35, 57, 58, 60, 61, 62, 65, 78, 79, 95, 99, 100, 126, 127, 129, 149, 153, 154, 158, 173, 174, 175, 176, 177, 212, 214
fibromyalgia · 17, 126, 127, 128, 129, 238
flexibility · 14, 96, 159, 173, 187, 189, 193
forced expiratory volume · 11, 40, 41, 83, 116, 234, 236
forced vital capacity · 11, 40, 41, 88, 116, 234, 236
fractures · 73, 190, 192, 231, 232

G

gaba · 12, 15, 44, 46, 61, 105, 146
gastroesophageal reflux · 131
gastrointestinal · 131, 153, 161, 169
generalized anxiety disorder · 34, 54
gerd · 131

H

hatha yoga · 14, 25, 43, 51, 52, 53, 73, 93, 102, 105, 111, 114, 127, 130, 132, 149, 157, 159, 165, 181, 193, 206, 229
headaches · 18, 169, 171, 172, 216, 239
heart failure · 17, 68, 69, 95, 96, 97, 98, 103, 133
heart rate variability[24] · 11
hippocampus · 12, 16, 104
hiv · 137, 139, 140, 141, 142, 238
hyperlipidemia · 219
hypertension · 11, 14, 80, 86, 91, 92, 133, 134, 135, 136, 137, 138, 139, 164, 194, 198, 202, 219, 226, 231

I

ibs · 153, 154, 155
immune · 17, 63, 67, 103, 115, 139, 141, 173, 175
Immune function · 12
immunity · 17, 147
incontinence · 157, 231, 232
infection · 139, 140, 141, 151, 202, 216
infertility · 143, 144, 145, 198
inflammation · 12, 17, 41, 86, 93, 94, 97, 115, 147, 181, 198, 199, 216
insomnia · 54, 56, 66, 99, 126, 147, 148, 149, 150, 158, 159, 160
insulin resistance · 106, 107, 109
Interstitial cystitis · 151, 152
Irritable bowel syndrome · 153, 154, 155
ischemic heart disease · 219

K

kripalu · 25, 111, 179, 181, 194, 206

L

lifestyle changes · 133, 164, 178
lipid · 11, 92

M

maximum voluntary ventilation · 11, 41, 88
mbrp · 112
mbsr · 140, 151, 152, 171, 199, 212
meditation · 10, 11, 12, 14, 15, 16, 17, 19, 20, 21, 22, 25, 29, 31, 32, 33, 35, 36, 37, 38, 53, 55, 56, 61, 63, 68, 70, 82, 91, 100, 104, 107, 123, 124, 125, 130, 135, 138, 142, 148, 150, 165, 167, 171, 172, 180, 184, 185, 214, 227, 235
melatonin · 12, 16, 147
memory · 30, 32, 78, 110, 126, 147, 195
menopause · 157, 159, 160, 181, 239
menorrhagia · 161
menstrual · 157, 161, 162, 198

N

O

191, 193, 197, 214, 215, 219, 220, 232, 233

94, 95, 96, 97, 98, 99, 100, 101, 102, 103, 104, 105, 107, 108, 109, 111, 112, 113, 114, 116, 117, 118, 119, 121, 122, 123, 124, 125, 127, 128, 129, 130, 132, 134, 135, 137, 138, 140, 141, 142, 144, 145, 146, 147, 148, 149, 150, 151, 152, 153, 154, 156, 157, 158, 159, 161, 162, 164, 165, 167, 168, 170, 171, 173, 174, 175, 176, 178, 179, 180, 181, 182, 183, 184, 186, 187, 188, 189, 191, 193, 194, 195, 196, 197, 198, 199, 200, 202, 203, 204, 205, 206, 208, 209, 213, 214, 215, 216, 219, 220, 221, 222, 224, 227, 228, 229, 230, 231, 233, 234, 235, 236, 252

About the Author

Dr. Agarwal is an Internist/Cardiologist with strong interest in Integrative Medicine. He has published yoga related articles in many national and international journals. He has also presented yoga related abstracts/posters at both national and international meetings. He may be reached at:

usacardiologist@gmail.com

www.ingramcontent.com/pod-product-compliance
Lightning Source LLC
Chambersburg PA
CBHW071253220526
45468CB00001B/114